Grey Cases For Paediatric Examinations

David J Field
DM FRCP (Ed) DCH
Senior Lecturer in Child Health
University of Leicester
Leicester, UK

John Stroobant
FRCP DCH
Consultant Paediatrician
Children's Hospital
Lewisham
London, UK

Alan Fenton
MD MRCP
Lecturer in Child Health
University of Leicester
Leicester Royal Infirmary
Leicester, UK

Ian Maconochie
MB BS MRCP (I)
Paediatric Registrar
Children's Hospital
Lewisham, UK

Christopher O'Callaghan
DM MRCP B Med Sci
Senior Lecturer in Child Health
University of Leicester
Honorary Consultant
Leicester Royal Infirmary
Leicester, UK

CHURCHILL LIVINGSTONE
EDINBURGH LONDON MADRID MELBOURNE NEW YORK AND TOKYO 1995

CHURCHILL LIVINGSTONE
Medical Division of Longman Group Limited

Distributed in the United States of America by Churchill
Livingstone Inc., 650 Avenue of the Americas, New York,
N.Y. 10011, and by associated companies, branches and
representives throughout the world.

First published 1995

ISBN 0 - 443 - 05011 - 2

British Library Cataloguing-in-Publication Data
A catalogue record for this book is available from the
British Library.

Library of Congress Cataloging-in-Publication Data
A catalog record for this book is available from the
Library of Congress.

The
publisher's
policy is to use
paper manufactured
from sustainable forestes

Produce by Longman Singapore Publishers (Pte) Ltd.,
Printed in Singapore

Grey Cases for Paediatric Examinations

Contents

Introduction

The MRCP (UK) paediatric examination is divided into two parts:

1. Part I — a multiple choice examination testing mainly the candidate's knowledge base;
2. Part II — a test of clinical abilities. The exam consists of written and clinical sections.

This book is intended to help candidates prepare for the written portion of Part II. The written section of the exam has three parts:

1. Questions based on a series of 20 clinical pictures presented in a book;
2. 10 items of clinical data to be interpreted;
3. 'Grey cases' (normally 5).

Each of these sections has equal weighting and marks are pooled to give each candidate a final score out of 20. Only those who achieve 9 or more are permitted to progress to the clinical.

This book contains 100 'grey cases' divided into 20 mock exams. In order to obtain most benefit we suggest that you set aside 55 minutes (the time allocated in the real examination) and complete all 5 cases before checking your answers.

There is an increasing tendency for the examiners to include additional clinical material within at least one of the 'grey cases' to produce a composite case history. This may take the form of X-rays, growth charts, pathology material, etc. We have tried to adopt this same style where appropriate.

Again in keeping with the real examination, normal ranges are not given for results of standard investigations but are included for more unusual tests.

It is uncommon to be able to reach a single conclusion for each grey case. You must use all the information provided and decide which is the most likely answer. However, responses should be as precise and as specific as possible and reflect the postgraduate nature of the examination. Do not use abbreviations.

In the real exam each of the cases will have been discussed and a hierarchy of answers worthy of marks determined. Similar decisions will have been reached about answers which are definitely wrong on the basis of the information given.

The actual marking of the MRCP (UK) exam is very precise. Each answer is marked by an examiner who is blind to everything about the candidate except his/her exam number. Each question is marked separately rather than examiners marking whole papers. Marks are awarded only for the predetermined correct answers. Candidates must therefore be very precise in their responses; avoid the temptation to add an explanation unless specifically requested and ensure the answer is legible. No negative marks are awarded and therefore all questions should be answered.

In constructing this material we have tried, where possible, to present answers in a graded fashion; answers of equal value are grouped, eg.:

trauma drug abuse	best answers
child abuse tuberculous meningitis	correct but less appropriate than above
metabolic disorder	least acceptable answer on basis of information given.

Where it seems appropriate specific wrong answers are also indicated. In order that you are unable to discount any diagnosis simply because it has' already appeared in the book we have allowed ourselves one or two 'repeats'.

Finally, perhaps the most useful advice in approaching the MRCP (UK) as a whole is to deal with the problems as you would in your day-to-day work. Where a diagnosis seems obvious or a simple investigation is required always choose this as opposed to something more esoteric.

Paper 1 *QUESTIONS*

Question 1.1

A 34-year-old caucasian woman delivered a 39-week-gestation boy weighing 2.76 kg by normal delivery. The midwife noticed that the infant appeared to have short limbs and therefore asked the paediatrician to see the baby.

This was the mother's second child; she had a daughter aged $2\frac{1}{2}$ years who was well. Both parents were healthy and lived together in their own home. The father worked in the leather industry and the mother was a housewife. The father had a mentally-handicapped brother but the cause of this was unkown.

During the pregnancy there were a number of problems. Throughout the first half, the baby's mother suffered frequent small vaginal blood loss. Ultrasound scan had shown no abnormality in the infant and a normally placed placenta. During the later stages of pregnancy, the mother was admitted on a number of occasions with abdominal pain and on one of these admissions, a urinary tract infection was confirmed and treated successfully. The onset of labour was spontaneous and there followed a rapid progression to a normal delivery.

On examination the baby was pink in air and was without respiratory distress. All four limbs were short but both hands and feet appeared normal, as shown below. The baby had a relatively broad forehead but otherwise facial features were unremarkable. The only other abnormality on examination was the absence of a red reflex in both eyes.

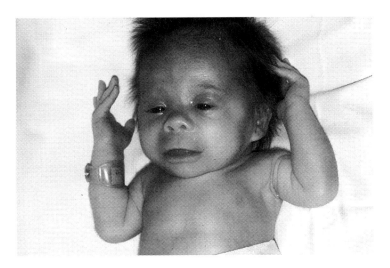

1. Suggest a diagnosis.
2. What three further investigations would you perform?

Question 1.2

A 5-year-old girl returned to the UK from the Middle East where she had been living for the past 4 years. During this time she experienced recurrent wheezy episodes and upper respiratory tract infections, intermittent diarrhoea and occasional herpes labialis infections and conjunctivitis. She had not been investigated in the past but was admitted to hospital on her return with another severe episode of conjunctivitis. Apart from an inflamed eye, physical examination was normal. Her weight was on the 3rd centile, and height on the 25th.

Haemoglobin	10.9 g/dl, normal film
White cell count	$8.3 \times 10^9/l$
Platelet count	$210 \times 10^9/l$
Urea and electrolytes	Normal
Sweat sodium	59 mmol/l
IgG	5.6 g/l (normal 5.6–14.9 g/l)
IgA	0.5 g/l (normal 0.5–2.2 g/l)
Chest X-ray	Normal
Pelvic X-ray	Normal
Liver function tests	Normal
Ferritin	Normal

1. What is the likely diagnosis?
2. What investigation would you perform to establish this diagnosis?
3. What is the treatment for this condition?

Question 1.3

A 9-week-old male caucasian infant was referred for investigation. He was the first child of healthy parents and was born at 37 weeks, labour being induced for maternal pre-eclampsia. His birthweight was 2.1 kg.

He initially went to the postnatal ward, but developed a distended abdomen on the second day of life, passing foul, blood-stained stools. He underwent laparotomy and an ileal perforation was found, requiring resection of 4 cm of bowel and the formation of a defunctioning ileostomy. The postoperative period was complicated by two brief generalized convulsions, treated with phenobarbitone, and paralytic ileus, requiring the use of total parenteral nutrition for 4 weeks. He also developed a heart murmur consistent with patent ductus arteriosus, although he was not clinically in heart failure. He was noted to be jaundiced on the third day of life and required a brief period of phototherapy. The jaundice was said to have fluctuated since that time. He had been breast fed at home. A cousin had cystic fibrosis.

On examination he looked thin (weight 3.5 kg) and was icteric. Pulse rate and character were within normal limits. He had a short systolic murmur in the pulmonary area. The liver margin was 3 cm below the costal margin and the spleen was just palpable. The ileostomy fluid was yellow.

INR	1.3
Total protein	53 g/l
Albumin	38 g/l
Alkaline phosphatase	386 IU/l (normal <350 IU/l)
Gamma glutamyl transferase	778 IU/l (normal 5–55 IU/l)
Alanine transaminase	160 IU/l (normal 2–53 IU/l)
Total bilirubin	140 µmol/l; 126 µmol/l direct
Abdominal ultrasound	Normal liver parenchyma, gallbladder visualized, no bile duct dilatation, spleen enlarged, kidneys normal
Chest X-ray	Normal cardiac contour, lung fields clear, butterfly vertebrae
Echocardiogram	Normal cardiac connections, no patent ductus arteriosus, peripheral pulmonary artery stenosis
Cardiac catheter:	
Right atrial pressure	9 mmHg (a wave), 5 mmHg (v wave)
Right ventricular pressure	60/5 mmHg
Main pulmonary artery pressure	60/5 mmHg
Distal pulmonary artery pressure	22/12 mmHg

There was no step up in oxygen saturation from right atrium to right ventricle to pulmonary artery.

1. Give four possible diagnoses.
2. What three investigations would you perform?

Question 1.4

A 13-year-old caucasian boy presented to the A&E department with a 10-day history of recurrent rectal bleeding. It was usually bright red, accompanied by diarrhoea, up to 7 times a day, but no mucus. There had been intermittent, colicky lower abdominal pain, his appetite had decreased and he had lost weight. He had been healthy in the past and his family was generally well. His parents had recently separated. He had last travelled about 2 years ago to the USA and Spain.

Examination on admission showed a pale boy of average height and weight. His temperature was 37.5°C, blood pressure 110/70 mmHg and pulse rate 80 beats/min. His abdomen was generally tender on palpation but there was no guarding and no localization. Examination was otherwise normal.

Haemoglobin	12.9 g/dl
White blood cells	6.5×10^9/l
Neutrophils	60%
Lymphocytes	30%
Platelet count	299 x 10^9/1
ESR	32 mm/h
Ferritin	39 µg/l (normal 15–300 µg/l)
Stool microscopy	Amoebic cysts but no erythrophagocytic forms
Stool culture	No growth
Stool occult blood	Positive
Urine culture	Negative
Abdominal ultrasound scan	Normal
C-reactive protein	Negative
Autoantibody screen	Negative
Liver function tests:	
Serum bilirubin	10 µmol/l
Aspartate transaminase	23 IU/l
Alanine transaminase	30 IU/l
Serum total protein	72 g/l
Serum albumin	41 g/l

1. What is the most likely diagnosis?
2. What procedure is indicated now?
3. What treatment would you give?

Question 1.5

A girl of Afro-Caribbean origin presented at 3 months of age with a history of vomiting for 2 days. She attended casualty 2 days prior to this consultation having had three loose stools and specimens were taken which were negative for bacterial and viral pathogens. The vomiting was not projectile or bile-stained and she had not had further loose motions. She was born at full term by forceps with a birthweight of 3.2 kg. She had been immunized against DPT and polio.

On examination she was >10% dehydrated, with reduced skin turgor, sunken fontanelle and eyes. Her systolic blood pressure was 60 mmHg and her pulse rate 160 beats/min, regular with a thready quality. Apart from these findings examination was unremarkable and she was apyrexial.

Haemoglobin	11.8 g/dl
White cell count	$8.7 \times 10^9/l$
Platelet count	$681 \times 10^9/l$
Serum sodium	127 mmol/l
Serum potassium	2.8 mmol/l
Serum urea	21.4 mmol/l
Serum creatinine	160 mmol/l
Serum protein	75 g/dl
Serum albumin	49 g/dl
Serum bicarbonate	34 mmol/l
Serum chloride	62 mmol/l
Arterial blood gas in air:	
pH	7.64
PaO_2	8.3 kPa
$PaCO_2$	4.1 kPa
Base excess	$+17.6$ mmol/l
Abdominal ultrasound	Normal

1. Suggest a diagnosis.
2. What two investigations should be performed?

Paper 1 *ANSWERS*

Answer 1.1

1. Conradi's syndrome — autosomal recessive type
Conradi's syndrome — rhizomelic form

Congenital dwarfism

Chromosomal disorder
Congenital infection

Reject: Intrauterine growth retardation

2. Peroxisomal enzyme studies (specific for Conradi's)
Skeletal survey
Cardiac ultrasound
Renal ultrasound
Eye opinion

Chromosomal analysis
Congenital infection screen
Renal function tests

Discussion

This child has dysmorphic features and the combination of proximal limb shortening and loss of the red reflex suggests Conradi's syndrome. The red reflex relies on the existence of a clear eye (cornea, lens and vitreous) plus a healthy choroid and retina. In Conradi's syndrome the red reflex is lost because of cataracts.

Confirmation of the diagnosis can only come from specific enzyme assay of platelets or cultured fibroblasts. These tests often take a long time to carry out. In the interim other tests (e.g. skeletal survey) are appropriate to look for other features associated with Conradi's and to confirm the absence of features of alternative diagnoses (e.g. fractures in severe osteogenesis imperfecta). X-ray appearances are particularly helpful with epiphysial stippling and vertical clefting of the vertebral bodies being characteristic of Conradi's.

Answer 1.2

1. IgG subclass deficiency
Immunodeficiency

Reject: Schwachman's Syndrome
Atopy

Allergy
Food allergy
Asthma
Recurrent infection
Malabsorbtion

2. IgG subclass estimation

3. Prophylactic antibiotics, e.g. cotrimoxazole
Regular intravenous immunoglobulin therapy

Physiotherapy

Discussion

The pointers to this girl's diagnosis include her recurrent episodes of wheeze, diarrhoea and infection. While simple asthma might account for some of her symptoms, her recurrent infections and diarrhoea are not typical of this. Food allergy might produce diarrhoea but not a recurrent herpes infection. Although not necessarily pathological, her weight on the 3rd centile suggests a degree of failure to thrive. Other explanations for her symptoms would include cystic fibrosis and Schwachman's syndrome. While failure to thrive with diarrhoea would explain both of these conditions, the sweat test is normal and the presence of normal chest and pelvic X-rays do not suggest Schwachman's syndrome; in this condition typically there is an abnormal gait because of metaphyseal achondroplasia. Furthermore, her white cell count is within normal limits and although this is an isolated finding from the data given, Schwachman's syndrome is not an appropriate conclusion.

Although the IgG and IgA are at the very bottom limit of normal, this is a typical finding in isolated IgG subclass deficiency. All of the features in the history are consistent with this, but unless IgG subclasses are looked for, the diagnosis will be missed. Therefore, it is essential to perform this particular investigation.

Many children with minor infections respond to prophylactic antibiotics and their condition often improves as they get older. If they continue to have recurrent episodes of infection, causing failure to thrive or other significant symptoms, then intravenous immunoglobulin therapy is necessary.

Other, non-specific answers are not appropriate. There is enough evidence from the data given that there is no malabsorption.

Answer 1.3

1. Alagille's syndrome
Extrahepatic biliary atresia
Hepatic dysfunction secondary to intravenous feeding
Cystic fibrosis

Reject: Hepatitis
             Breast-milk jaundice

2. Liver isotope excretion scan (e.g. HIDA)
    Liver biopsy (to exclude biliary atresia)
    Ophthalmological examination (posterior embryotoxin)
    Sweat test

Reject: Rose–Bengal test

Discussion

The patient has Alagille's syndrome (biliary hypoplasia, arteriohepatic dysplasia), suggested by the combination of hyperbilirubinaemia and vertebral and cardiac anomalies. The aetiology of this condition is unknown, although familial cases (15% of the total) have suggested both autosomal dominant (with variable expression) and recessive modes of inheritance. 20% are born preterm or small for gestational age. The majority of cases are sporadic and teratogens such as congenital viral infections have been suggested as a cause. Chronic cholestasis is usually the dominant clinical problem, although 10% may have cyanotic heart disease. Cardiac anomalies occur in up to 95% of cases, peripheral pulmonary artery stenosis being a common finding (50%). Other common extrahepatic features include posterior embryotoxon (70%, seen on slit-lamp examination), skeletal anomalies (50%, butterfly vertebrae) and abnormal facies. Renal, neural and endocrine anomalies together with delayed mental and sexual development have also been described. A liver biopsy is essential in cases presenting in infancy (although pathological changes are often difficult to identify), to exclude biliary atresia. Up to 90% of cases present with a hepatitis syndrome.

Extrahepatic biliary atresia must be considered in any child presenting with persisting conjugated hyperbilirubinaemia, since early surgical drainage by hepatic portoenterostomy can reduce morbidity and mortality. The identification of a gallbladder on ultrasound does not exclude the condition, diagnosis being made using a combination of ultrasound, isotope excretion scan (the Rose–Bengal test is no longer used) and liver biopsy.

Hepatic dysfunction has been described following intravenous feeding for periods of 10–180 days, being commoner in sick preterm babies and neonates with surgical problems. The aetiology is unknown and all the main components of intravenous feeding have been implicated as causative factors. The incidence increases with prematurity, the duration of intravenous feeding and the persistent absence of oral feeding. The hepatic dysfunction gradually remits over about 6 months since total parenteral feeding is discontinued, with liver biopsy changes persisting for up to 1 year. Progression to cirrhosis inevitably occurs if intravenous feeding has to be continued.

Prolonged conjugated hyperbilirubinaemia in infants is rare as a presenting feature of cystic fibrosis.

Answer 1.4

1. Inflammatory bowel disease
  Ulcerative colitis
  Crohn's disease

  Infective gastroenteritis
  Peptic ulceration
  Intussusception
  Meckel's diverticulum

Reject: Rectal polyp
       Anal fissure

2. Colonoscopy with bowel biopsies
  Sigmoidoscopy

  Barium enema
  Barium meal with follow through

3. Trial of oral metronidazole
  Systemic steroids
  Mesalazine or sulphasalazine
  Correction of fluid, electrolyte and albumin deficits
  Steroid enemas
  Nutritional support

  Surgical correction of polyps

  H_2 blockers and antacids for peptic ulceration

Discussion

Ulcerative colitis is the most likely explanation in the absence of an apparent infective cause (although this still remains a possibility), as the stool culture is negative and amoebiasis is excluded by the absence of erythrophagocytic forms of amoebae. The ESR is slightly raised, consistent with ulcerative colitis rather than Crohn's disease. The low normal ferritin (in this age group) is consistent with chronic blood loss. The history is not entirely compatible with a Meckel's diverticulum or intussusception (and is rare at this age). Although bright red bleeding is possible with peptic ulceration, the history of diarrhoea is against this. A polyp or a fissure is unlikely to produce such pain, anaemia and weight loss.

It is important to confirm the presence of colitis both microscopically and by histology. This is most appropriately done by colonoscopy and biopsy. Barium studies are less important at this stage unless the histology is normal. Clearly the barium enema must in any case precede the barium meal.

Treatment will depend on the final diagnosis. An initial trial of metronidazole may be justified in the first instance if the patient is not toxic and there is doubt about the exclusion of an infective cause. Current treatment advice for both ulcerative colitis and Crohn's disease involves the use of steroids and sulphasalazine. Rarely, surgical resection may be indicated.

Answer 1.5

1. Bartter's syndrome

Cystic fibrosis

Thiazide abuse

Dehydration

Reject: Pyloric stenosis
Congenital adrenal hyperplasia

2. Serum renin level
Sweat test
Thiazide level

Discussion

Causes of metabolic alkalosis with low serum sodium, potassium and chloride include increased gastric loss such as with pyloric stenosis, gastric drainage without electrolyte replacement, the use of thiazide diuretics, Bartter's syndrome and cystic fibrosis. The history is suggestive of acute dehydration with the symptoms being disproportionately less severe than the signs. As the likelihood of viral or bacterial pathogens is small and there is no persistent diarrhoea, other causes need to be considered.

Severe salt depletion with mild gastrointestinal disorder is a well recognized mode of presentation of cystic fibrosis, but cystic fibrosis is rare in Afro-Caribbeans. The more likely diagnosis is Bartter's syndrome, which is characterized by hypertrophy of the juxta-glomerular apparatus with hyperaldosteronism, elevated renin, a decreased response to angiotensin-2 and hypokalaemic alkalosis. Tubular proteinuria, decreased renal concentrating ability and sodium loss in the urine are noted features. Administration of thiazide diuretics as a presentation of Meadow's syndrome (Munchausen by proxy) or child abuse is a remote possibility, but does not tie in with the diarrhoeal component of the illness. Pyloric stenosis is rejected as there is no palpable tumour. Congenital adrenal hyperplasia is rejected as the chloride concentration is very low.

Paper 2 *QUESTIONS*

Question 2.1

A 5-month-old boy of Asian parents was reviewed on the paediatric ward. He had been admitted 3 weeks earlier with a history of breathlessness, cough and temperature. During that admission he had been shown to have a large left-sided pleural effusion. He was treated with antibiotics and the effusion tapped revealed straw-coloured fluid. Within 48 h he showed signs of improvement and therefore was allowed home.

The boy was born in the UK, the product of a normal pregnancy and delivery. He was given BCG at birth. Apart from his recent illness he had been completely well. The parents shared their house where six adults and five children lived. Both parents were well and were first cousins. They worked for the family textile business.

At the review, the parents reported that they had noticed a gradual return of breathlessness and intermittent fever; they had recorded temperatures up to 38.5°C. There was a BCG scar in the region of the left deltoid. Cardiovascular examination was normal except that the apex beat could not be located. In the respiratory system there was a dullness to percussion and diminished breath sounds over a large portion of the left chest. Examination of the abdomen was limited since the child had recently been fed and there was fairly marked gaseous distension. Neurologically, the child appeared normal.

1. Suggest two diagnoses to explain the pleural effusion.
2. Give four investigations you would perform.

Question 2.2

A $2\frac{1}{2}$-year-old boy who had previously been well presented with a 3-day history of vomiting, variable drowsiness and a 2-min generalized convulsion, which started with a left-sided clonic movement and rapidly progressed to involve both sides of his body. He had had one febrile convulsion in the past but on this occasion he was afebrile. His birth and development were normal; he had had no other serious illness subsequently.

His mother was well although she had recently had an herpetic lesion on her lip and the boy's younger sister had an upper respiratory tract infection. His father had no contact with the family.

On examination the boy was drowsy but rousable; Glasgow coma score was 13. His temperature was 37.8°C, pulse 110 beats/min, respiratory rate 20 breaths/min and blood pressure 100/70 mmHg. Pupils were equal and reacting directly and consensually. Fundoscopy was normal. His cranial nerves were normal. There was slightly increased tone in the left arm and leg with increased reflexes and an equivocal plantar response. Reflexes were normal on the right with a normal plantar response. Physical examination was otherwise normal. An EEG was performed which showed the following record:

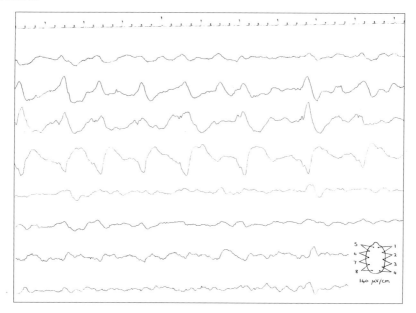

1. What two further investigations would you perform?
2. What three therapeutic steps would you take?
3. What is the most likely diagnosis?

After 2 days of treatment, his conscious level improved for 24 h (Glasgow coma score 14), but he deteriorated again with a Glasgow coma score of 10.

4. What is the diagnosis?

Question 2.3

A 9-year-old girl was admitted for investigation of mild exertional dyspnoea and cyanosis. She had had extrahepatic biliary atresia treated with Kasai portoenterostomy at the age of 7 weeks. Following this, although she had remained jaundiced, her liver function had been stable, her stools were described as containing some pigment and she had had no episodes of cholangitis. Her growth and development were satisfactory. She was also known to have left isomerism and ventricular septal defect, the latter being felt to be closing spontaneously. A cardiac catheter performed in infancy showed the pulmonary artery pressure to be approximately one-third of systemic pressure.

On examination she was jaundiced and centrally cyanosed, with several spider naevi. She was appropriately grown for her age. Her respiratory rate at rest was 25 breaths/min and her chest was clear. There was a 3/6 systolic murmur heard best at the left sternal edge. Her liver was firm and palpable 4 cm below the costal margin.

Haemoglobin	12.2 g/dl
White cell count	5.5×10^9/l
Platelet count	149×10^9/l
INR	1.1
Albumin	44 g/l
Alkaline phosphatase	584 IU/l (normal <350 IU/l)
Gamma glutamyl tranferase	274 IU/l (normal 5–55 IU/l)
Alanine transferase	88 IU/l (normal 2–53 IU/l)
Total bilirubin	127 µmol/l; 107 µmol/l direct
ECG	Superior QRS axis, no ventricular hypertrophy
Cardiac catheter:	
Right ventricular pressure	22/0 mmHg
Main pulmonary artery pressure	22/15 mmHg

There was no step up in oxygen saturation from right atrium to right ventricle to pulmonary artery.

1. Suggest a diagnosis.
2. What two investigations would you perform to establish this diagnosis?
3. What therapeutic option is available for this patient?

Question 2.4

A 5-year-old boy was referred because his speech had deteriorated at the age of 4 years 3 months. Prior to this age he could converse freely with adults about events and talk on the telephone using normal vocabulary and grammar. In the 3 months before his speech deteriorated, there had been a number of stressful family events, including the death of his grandfather. Over a period of a few days it was noticed that he started mumbling and ignoring people who spoke to him. His hearing was formally checked at this time and found to be normal. He started making sounds like words but which were not words. However, he played with toys appropriately and looked at faces and was aware of speech but gave no response to verbal labels for objects. A febrile convulsion had been diagnosed when he was 4 years old. Another short seizure occurred 6 months later. The parents, reassured by the benign nature of his first fit, did not seek medical help. He had no other obvious neurological problem. CT and MRI scans of his head were normal.

With counselling and psychiatric help, his behaviour improved but his speech did not return. The child appeared bewildered when spoken to and looked blank. Over the next 2 years, without psychiatric intervention, there was gradual improvement in the child's aphasia. Repeated audiological investigations showed no abnormality.

1. What is the most likely diagnosis?
2. What investigations will help to confirm your diagnosis?

Question 2.5

A 40-week-gestation boy, birthweight 3.3 kg, was delivered by routine caesarian section for cephalopelvic disproportion. The antenatal course had been quite normal.

Grunting and tachypnoea developed 30 min after delivery and a non-specific erythematous rash appeared on the upper part of the baby's trunk. His initial BM stix was 6 mmol/l. His chest X-ray was noted to be hazy. An arterial blood gas sample taken from the right radial artery revealed:

pH   7.17
PaO_2 8.7 kPa
$PaCO_2$ 7.7 kPa
HCO_3 17 mmol/l in air

He was therefore intubated and ventilated and given two doses of surfactant via the endotracheal tube. Full septic screen, including lumbar puncture, blood cultures and skin swabs were taken and he was started on intravenous antibiotics.

At 18 hours of age he was noted to be developing mottling of his lower limbs and had a poor urine output of <1 ml/kg/h. An arterial blood gas at that time was:

pH   7.18
PaO_2 10.9 kPa
$PaCO_2$ 3.2 kPa
HCO_3 16 mmol/l

His ventilator settings were 60 breaths/min, inspiratory pressure 25 mmHg, expiratory pressure 3 mmHg, inspired fraction of oxygen 80%. Pulse oximetry on his left big toe fluctuated between 75% and 95% saturated.

On examination, the child appeared slightly jaundiced. He had a cleft palate. Cardiovascular auscultation revealed first and second heart sounds to be present but difficult to hear because of the ventilator. A continuous murmur was heard intermittently between his scapulae. His abdominal examination revealed a 2-cm liver. The central nervous system was difficult to assess as the child was sedated.

1. What two further signs should be sought?
2. What investigations should be performed?
3. What treatment should be commenced?

Paper 2 *ANSWERS*

Answer 2.1

1. Infection
Post-infection
Malignancy

Reject: Chylothorax
Heart failure

2. Pleural tap
Pleural fluid for microscopy and culture (including tuberculosis)
Pleural fluid for measurement of protein content
Pleural fluid for cytology
Chest and abdominal CT scan
Abdominal ultrasound
Chest ultrasound
Mantoux 1 in 10 000

Chest X-ray
Full blood count
C-reactive protein
ESR
Viral titres

Echocardiogram

Discussion

This child has symptoms and signs suggestive of a recurrent effusion in the left chest. There is little in the information provided to aid in forming a diagnosis. The child's race and overcrowded living conditions suggest a predisposition to tuberculosis; however, BCG had been given which reduces, but does not exclude, this possibility. The fact the parents are first cousins is unlikely to have any significance in these circumstances.

Given the information, the two most likely diagnosis are infection or malignant disease. A low-grade fever might result from either condition. In reality the failure to complete an examination of the abdomen was a serious omission since on ultrasound a mass was identified in the abdomen and extension into the chest was confirmed by CT. Open biopsy was performed and confirmed a diagnosis of neuroblastoma. Urine catecholamine estimation would have been an appropriate test but this conclusion is not really possible from the information given.

Answer 2.2

1. OCT scan
MRI scan
Viral titres (specifically herpetic)
Paul–Bunnell test/monospot

Blood culture

2. Intravenous acyclovir (500 mg/m^2 t.d.s. for 10/7)
Intravenous mannitol
Fluid restriction to two-thirds of maintenance
Steroids

Start anticonvulsants

3. Right parietal herpes simplex encephalitis
Right parietal encephalitis

Encephalitis

Tumour or space-occupying lesion

Reject: Meningitis
Metabolic disorder

4. Relapsing herpes simplex encephalitis

Bleed into tumour

Discussion

The clues to the diagnosis are the EEG — which shows quite clearly a very high voltage (140 µV/cm) in the right parietal area — and the maternal herpetic lesion. The EEG disturbance has both the characteristics of an encephalitis and a site which is typical of herpes simplex.

The site of the lesion can be confirmed on CT or MRI scan. To confirm the diagnosis of the herpes simplex a Paul–Bunnell or monospot test is useful to exclude other causes or encephalitis. Blood culture might be useful, but is not the most important investigation to establish the diagnosis, given the abnormal EEG.

The treatment for this condition is intravenous acyclovir. Alteration in conscious level may be partially or completely reversed by the use of intravenous mannitol. Similarly, the use of fluid restriction may also improve the cerebral oedema. Because of his previous convulsion and current condition, the use of anticonvulsants is helpful. Steroids may have a place in the presence of a space-occupying lesion and in relapsing herpes simplex encephalitis.

With this characteristic EEG there is little else that explains the pathology, although the presence of a tumour or space-occupying lesion in the parietal region might produce such an abnormality. The initial improvement followed by further deterioration is consistent with the development of a relapsing herpes simplex encephalitis, which has a particularly poor outcome. In this situation further acyclovir and steroids may be useful. However, it has been suggested that anti-inflammatory treatment, e.g. with cyclophosphamide, may also be useful, particularly when there is evidence of viral replication during this relapsing phase. Were there a tumour or space-occupying lesion present, this deterioration could be explained by haemorrhage within it.

Answer 2.3

1. Right-to-left shunt (non-cardiac)
Multiple peripheral pulmonary arteriovenous fistulae
Arteriovenous malformation

Reject: Eisenmenger's syndrome

2. Echocardiogram
Cardiac catheterization with pulmonary angiography

3. Liver transplantation

Discussion

The history suggests a right-to-left shunt. The absence of respiratory signs makes primary pulmonary pathology unlikely. Patients with chronic hepatic dysfunction are at risk of developing pulmonary arteriovenous fistulae which can result in hypoxaemia. Although their exact aetiology is uncertain, they may result either from a failure of hepatic synthetic function or from hepatic metabolic failure (e.g. failure to remove circulating oestrogens). The same mechanism is thought to be responsible for the formation of spider naevi. Multiple lesions in the periphery of the lung will result in right-to-left shunting and cyanosis, which may become more marked on exertion. Pulmonary angiography may reveal a single large malformation, or if there are multiple small lesions, contrast will appear very rapidly in the left-sided atrium. A further diagnostic refinement would be to perform echocardiography (preferably transoesophageal) using echo contrast (to produce microbubbles) injected into the pulmonary artery. In the presence of intrapulmonary shunts the contrast will appear in the left-sided atrium. Liver transplantation and restoration of normal liver function may cause the regression of these shunts in a proportion of patients. Transplantation may have to be performed even if (as in this case) liver function is adequate, since otherwise the shunts become increasingly significant and eventually the degree of hypoxaemia may preclude transplantation.

The past history of a ventricular septal defect raises the possibility of pulmonary vascular disease and Eisenmenger's syndrome, but the previous catheter data do not support this. Echocardiography will indicate whether the defect has closed, and which ventricle appears dominant. A further indication of the relative ventricular pressures may be obtained if the defect has closed spontaneously with the formation of a pseudoaneurysm, since the latter will bow out towards the side of lowest pressure.

Since this patient has left isomerism, a further possibility is anomalous systemic venous return. This, however, would give rise to persistent cyanosis and would have been detected at the time of previous cardiac catheterization.

Answer 2.4

1. Landau–Kleffner syndrome

Psychiatric problem/illness/reaction
Minor motor status/other forms of epilepsy
Chronic lead poisoning

2. EEG

Discussion

Landau–Kleffner syndrome is a rare disorder and needs differentiation from psychiatric illness, deafness and progressive neurodegenerative disease. The clinical picture is often quite dramatic when a child who has developed speech and language normally suffers an abrupt or gradual loss of speech. In some cases, at the same time or shortly afterwards, generalized or focal motor type seizures may develop. The age of onset of the disorder is between 3 and 9 years and the course is variable. The aetiology remains obscure.

Deafness has been excluded as a cause by normal audiological investigation and the history is not typical of another form of epilepsy. A psychological reaction is the most likely of the differential diagnoses.

The development of mutism is one of the few indications for a standard EEG in an apparently psychiatric disorder. In this case the EEG showed frequent bursts of spike and wave recurring throughout the recording with a frequency of 2–3 Hz and a generalized distribution. This, together with the classical case history, confirmed the diagnosis.

Answer 2.5

1. Presence and characteristics of femoral pulses
Four-limb blood pressure measurement

2. Echocardiogram
Electrocardiogram
Aortic angiography

3. Intravenous prostaglandin
Correction of acidosis
Use of intravenous ionotropes

Discussion

This child has mottling of the lower limbs and a poor urinary output. These are indirect indicators of an inadequate systemic circulation. He also has tachypnoea, an enlarged liver and a continuous murmur (the latter typical of a patent arterial duct). These, with the hazy chest X-ray, are indicative of heart failure in the neonate. The clinical picture suggests a duct-dependent cardiac lesion with variable duct patency. In particular, the systemic circulation is impaired.

Obstruction of aortic blood flow may be caused by lesions such as aortic stenosis or coarctation of the aorta. Reduced systemic blood flow may also result from poor ventricular function.

Patent ductus arteriosus closure in this setting is a medical emergency and prostaglandin should be given to maintain patency. The use of bicarbonate will temporarily relieve the acidosis and lower pulmonary artery pressure. The use of ionotropes may improve the circulation for a short period, but corrective surgery will be required.

Paper 3 *QUESTIONS*

Question 3.1

A midwife arranged for the admission of a 2-week-old baby whom she had noticed to have a swollen and erythematous left arm.

The baby had been a normal delivery at term weighing 3.65 kg. There had been some concern in the last week of pregnancy because of poor fetal movements and therefore labour had been induced. Labour progressed uneventfully and Apgar scores were 8 at 1 min and 9 at 5 min. The child's father was a policeman and his mother a physical education teacher. Both were in excellent health. This was their first child.

On examination the child looked healthy and was apyrexial. The infant was quiet and made few spontaneous movements, although fine jerks of the fingers were noted. The left arm was reddened and a little swollen, but the child's mother felt that the changes were becoming less obvious. The arm was not tender and had a full range of movement. The child was very alert but his tone was generally reduced. There were no other abnormalities.

1. What is the diagnosis?
2. Give two investigations you should perform?

Question 3.2

A 13-year-old Nigerian boy was admitted to hospital for investigation of two episodes of bilateral carpopedal spasm which had occurred on the day of admission. Each lasted 5 min. Three days before this he had developed fever with a sore throat. He was otherwise well and had had no serious illnesses in the past. Physical examination showed him to be febrile with a temperature of 37.8°C and an inflamed throat. There was a positive Chvostek's sign.

Haemoglobin	11.5 g/dl
White cell count	4.3 × 10⁹/l
Platelet count	121 × 10⁹/l
ESR	20 mm/h
Sickle cell screen	Negative
Calcium	1.3 mmol/l (normal 2.2–2.8 mmol/l)
Alkaline phosphatase	181 IU/l (normal 30–250 IU/l)
Phosphate	2.69 mmol/l (normal 1.15–1.90 mmol/l)
Albumin	32 g/l
Magnesium	0.81 mmol/l (normal 0.6–0.95 mmol/l)
Bicarbonate	29 mmol/l
Parathyroid hormone	5 ng/l (normal 10–65 ng/l)

| Auto-antibody screen | Negative |
| Chest X-ray | Normal |

1. What is the diagnosis?
2. What two other tests for endocrine function would you perform to confirm the diagnosis?

Question 3.3

A boy was born at 38-weeks gestation to a single 18-year-old West Indian woman. His birthweight was 2.7 kg. The delivery was precipitate and the mother was unfortunately unattended at the moment of delivery. The midwifery staff returned to the delivery room approximately 2 min following delivery to find the infant pale and hypotonic. He had poor respiratory effort with a heart rate of 100 beats/min. The infant's colour improved rapidly following bag and mask resuscitation (Apgar 8 at 5 min), but he remained hypotonic and was therefore transferred to the neonatal unit. This was his mother's first pregnancy and it had been unremarkable apart from slightly reduced fetal movements.

Examination at the time of admission revealed a slightly dysmorphic infant who was markedly hypotonic. General systemic examination was otherwise unremarkable apart from bilateral undescended testes. His head circumference was 37 cm. His condition remained stable but the hypotonicity persisted and he required tube feeding.

Cranial ultrasound	No intraventricular haemorrhage, normal parenchyma
Ophthalmological examination	Normal
Hearing screen	Normal
TORCH screen	Normal
Creatine kinase	Normal
Serum and urine amino acids	Normal
Thyroid function	Normal
EMG	Normal
EEG	Normal
Chromosomal analysis	46 XY

His feeding gradually improved and he was discharged home at 3 weeks of age. He maintained appropriate weight gain and head circumference growth. At the age of 4 months his tone was improving apart from poor head control. He was described as a placid infant.

1. Suggest a cause for this infant's condition.
2. What further investigation would you perform?

Question 3.4

A tall 11-year-old child developed a limp with pain in the groin and knee. She was otherwise healthy and was in the school athletics team for high jump. She had an episode of tonsillitis 1 month prior to her hip pain developing. There were no associated bowel or bladder problems.

On examination she was apyrexial and there was no evidence of tenderness or swelling. As well as an obvious limp, abduction, internal rotation and flexion of the hip were limited. External rotation of the hip was noted with flexion. Careful measurement showed light limb shortening on the affected side. An X-ray of her hips and pelvis showed no obvious abnormality.

Haemoglobin	12.7 g/dl
White cell count	7.4×10^9/l
Platelet count	300×10^9/l
ESR	2
C-reactive protein	1 mg/dl
Rheumatoid factor	Negative
Anti-nuclear antibody	Negative

1. What is the most likely diagnosis?
2. What investigation is needed?

Question 3.5

A 3-year-old girl presented with a history of recurrent infections over the past 15 months. She had had six episodes of upper respiratory tract infections and three bouts of tonsillitis. The first episode of tonsillitis responded to antibiotic treatment but the later episodes responded less well, according to her mother. Over the past fortnight she had become pale and tired. She also complained of pains in her legs and bruised easily.

She was born at term weighing 3.2 kg by vaginal delivery and was fully immunized. She had reached her developmental milestones at the appropriate times but was below the 3rd centile for height and weight. She was not taking any medicines and had not had any contact with any toxins or chemicals. She was an only child; her father was a 42-year-old accountant and her mother a 38-year-old buyer for a clothing retailing company.

On examination she was irritable and pale with lesions on her leg (see picture overleaf). There were no petechiae or other skin lesions. She was coryzal and had enlarged tonsils. There was no lymphadenopathy, hepatomegaly or splenomegaly. Her fundi were normal and general examination was unremarkable apart from strabismus and shortened thumbs.

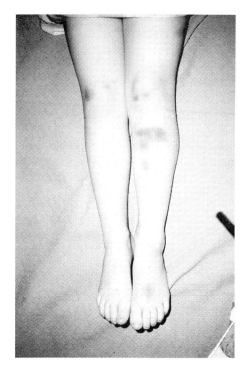

Haemoglobin	4.6 g/dl
White cell count	$3.4 \times 10^9/l$
Platelet count	$7.0 \times 10^9/l$
Blood film	Macrocytosis; mild poikilocytosis
Serum sodium	139 mmol/l
Serum potassium	3.9 mmol/l
Serum urea	3.4 mmol/l
Serum creatinine	40 mmol/l

1. What is the haematological picture?
2. What two investigations would you perform?
3. What is the diagnosis?

Paper 3 *ANSWERS*

Answer 3.1

1. Werdnig–Hoffman disease (anterior horn cell disease)

Congenital peripheral neuropathy

Osteomyelitis

Reject: Child abuse
            Dystrophia myotonica
            Congenital myopathy

2. Electromyography
Nerve conduction velocity
Muscle biopsy
Sural nerve biopsy
Blood cultures

X-ray of left arm
Creatine kinase

Full blood count
C-reactive protein

Discussion

This child has Werdnig–Hoffman disease (infantile anterior horn cell disease). The redness and swelling arise because he is unable to free his arm once he has been placed on his side. The lack of movement and fasciculation (fine finger jerks) are typical. Fasciculation is often most apparent in the tongue.

Differentiation from congenital peripheral neuropathy requires careful investigation with electromyography, nerve conduction studies and nerve and muscle biopsies. Congenital myopathy does not normally cause such profound weakness. Congenital myotonic dystrophy is unlikely with both parents well, especially as the mother is so physically fit.

Osteomyelitis is unlikely on the basis of the information given but cannot be safely excluded. Where doubt exists, cultures must be performed and antibiotics commenced.

Answer 3.2

1. Hypoparathyroidism
Autoimmune hypoparathyroidism

Reject: Hyperventilation
             Rickets

2. Thyroid function
   Serum cortisol
   Urinary calcium
   Vitamin D level

Discussion

This boy has hypocalcaemia. His high phosphate distinguishes hypoparathyroidism as a cause from rickets where there would normally be a low serum phosphate concentration. Similarly a normal phosphate concentration would indicate calciopenic rickets. However, in this situation there would be an elevated alkaline phosphatase and an abnormal X-ray. Both of these are normal in this boy. Futhermore the parathyroid hormone level is low, pointing to abnormal parathyroid function.

The usual explanation for hypoparathyroidism at this age is an autoimmune process and therefore this is the more precise answer. There is no suggestion from the physical examination that he has any of the features of the di George syndrome or pseudohypoparathyroidism. In the latter condition there are characteristic face and skeletal problems and in the former there is also associated immune deficiency.

Patients with autoimmune hypoparathyroidism may have other associated endocrine abnormalities, in particular Addison's disease and hypothyroidism. Both of these should be excluded. The treatment of this boy would include calcium and vitamin D.

Answer 3.3

1. Prader–Willi syndrome
   Non-specific mental retardation
   Benign congenital hypotonia

Reject: Spinal muscular dystrophy
             Congenital myotonic dystrophy
             Motor neuropathy

2. Detailed chromosomal analysis

Discussion

The first question to address in the assessment of a 'floppy' infant is whether there is associated muscular weakness. This is found in disorders such as hereditary infantile spinal muscular atrophy (Werdnig–Hoffman disease and other benign variants), congenital myopathies – both structural (central core disease and myotubular myopathies) and metabolic (glycogenoses types II and III, lipid storage myopathies, periodic paralysis), congenital myotonic and muscular dystrophies, motor neuropathies and neonatal myasthenia.

The infant's problem is profound hypotonia, which initially gave the impression of weakness. Conditions presenting in this way include those affecting the central nervous system (cerebral palsy, non-specific mental retardation, intrapartum trauma and asphyxia, intracranial haemorrhage, trisomy 21, organic and amino acidurias, sphingolipidoses, acute sepsis); those affecting connective tissue (congenital ligamentous laxity, Ehlers–Danlos syndrome, Marfan's syndrome, osteogenesis imperfecta, mucopolysaccharidoses); metabolic/endocrine disorders (renal tubular acidosis, hypercalcaemia, rickets, hypothyroidism); and others such as benign congenital hypotonia and Prader–Willi syndrome.

The diagnosis of Prader–Willi syndrome is suggested by the combination of hypotonia with poor sucking, gradually improving with age, dysmorphic facies (characteristically dolichocephaly, almond-shaped eyes, narrow face, small mouth with down-turned corners) and genital hypoplasia. There may be a history of poor fetal movement.

Diagnosis may be made by detailed chromosomal analysis. A deletion within bands 11–13 of the long arm (q) of chromosome 15 has been described in 50–75% of cases of Prader–Willi syndrome, and this deletion invariably occurs in the paternally-derived chromosome. Other infants who have the clinical syndrome may lack this particular cytogenetic deletion, of whom approximately 4% will have some other rearrangement involving the proximal segment of chromosome 15. The rest appear cytogenetically normal but 20% have been shown to have maternal uniparental disomy (i.e. both chromosomes being maternally derived).

Answer 3.4

1. Slipped capital femoral epiphysis
2. Frog-legged lateral view of the hips

Discussion

This child has a characteristic history and physical examination of a slipped capital femoral epiphyses. She was apyrexial and well with a normal ESR and C-reactive protein, making infection, malignancy and a connective tissue abnormality less likely.

Slipped capital femoral epiphysis is a disorder of the growth plate that occurs near the age of skeletal maturity. It involves an anterior, lateral and superior displacement of the metaphysis. The femur is thus externally rotated from under the epiphysis. Clinical presentation varies with the acuteness of the process. Most children present with a limp and varying degrees of ache or pain. The common presentation is discomfort in the groin, which is often referred to the knee. The paradoxical distribution of pain is attributed to referral within the femoral nerve distribution, which involves the hip and knee joints. Other patients have a very acute presentation of severe pain and inability to walk or move the hip.

A frog-legged lateral view of the hips is essential as slipped upper femoral epiphyses can easily be missed on an anteroposterior film. The earliest findings radiographically in patients with slipped femoral epiphysis are widening and irregularity of the growth plate and osteopenia of the femur. Later there is displacement of the epiphysis and avascular necrosis of the epiphysis or joint-space narrowing.

Answer 3.5

1. Pancytopenia

Reject: Anaemia
            Idiopathic thrombocytopenia

2. Bone marrow biopsy/trephine
   Chromosomal analysis

   Viral titres: parvovirus, Epstein-Barr virus, hepatitis A
   Urinary catecholamine assay

3. Fanconi's pancytopenia
   Aplastic anaemia (idiopathic)
   Leukaemia

   Neuroblastoma
   Viral-induced bone marrow suppression

Reject: Anaemia
            Idiopathic thrombocytopenia

Discussion

The results of the investigations show a pancytopenia with a macrocytosis and poikilocytosis revealing bone marrow dysfunction. Bone marrow infiltration may be caused by neuroblastoma or other malignancies such as leukaemia and should be considered in the differential diagnosis, hence the need for bone marrow sampling. Urinary catecholamine levels should be measured to diagnose neuroblastoma. Bone marrow suppression may be due to viral agents such as parvovirus, hepatitis A and Epstein-Barr virus and serial viral titres should be measured. However, these diagnoses are not associated with the skeletal or central nervous abnormalities mentioned.

This girl has the features of short stature and an aplastic anaemia. She also has skeletal abnormalities and stabismus; all these are seen in Fanconi's pancytopenia. Chromosomal analysis will show a high percentage of chromatin breaks and gaps.

Paper 4 *QUESTIONS*

Question 4.1

A baby was admitted to the neonatal unit at 48 h of age because of breathlessness. Pregnancy and labour had been unremarkable with rapid progression to a vertex delivery. Apgar scores were 9 at 1 min and 10 at 5 min and he had gone immediately to the breast. On the postnatal ward he had initially fed well but had become increasingly lethargic. He was the second child of healthy parents. His older sister had asthma but was otherwise well.

At the time of admission his respiratory rate was 100 breaths/min but he showed little or no recession. He was pale and irritable when disturbed. Blood pressure in the right arm was 76/50 mmHg. He was noted to pass urine with a good stream. A blood glucose was found to be 2.2 mmol/l. A blood gas analysis was performed on a sample from the right radial artery whilst the child was in air:

pH	7.1
PaO_2	11 kPa
$PaCO_2$	1.9 kPa
Base excess	−23 mmol/l

The chest X-ray was normal.

1. What is the diagnosis?
2. Give three investigations you should perform.

Question 4.2

A 4-year-old girl was referred by her GP for investigation of weight loss, despite a normal appetite. Her parents had not noted any other symptoms.

On examination she had an enlarged smooth thyroid gland. Her weight was on the 25th centile and height on the 75th. There was no lid lag but there was proptosis.

T4	235 nmol/l (normal 70–180 nmol/l)
TSH	0.1 µU/l (normal 0.25–5 µU/l)
Antithyroid antibodies	Positive 1 in 1000
Bone age	4 years

1. What is the diagnosis?
2. What treatment would you give?

3 years after finishing treatment she presented again to her GP with tiredness and slow growth. Her weight was on the 10th centile and height on the 25th.

T4	14.5 nmol/l
TSH	5.3 µU/l
Bone age	5 years

3. What is the diagnosis?
4. What treatment would you start?

Question 4.3

A 5-month-old caucasian boy was admitted following a 'funny turn'. He was picked up out of his cot that morning and his arms and shoulders appeared to twitch for a few seconds. Following this he did not respond in his usual way for about 30 min, but since that time he had been normal. His mother said he was "slow to breathe" at birth and he was admitted to the neonatal unit for 2 days, during which time no active treatment was required. His development since then had been normal. There was a family history of febrile convulsions.

Examination revealed a happy, alert, apyrexial infant, with weight and length on the 50th centile. The boy's head circumference was on the 97th centile and the anterior fontanelle was patent. Blood pressure was 170 mmHg systolic in all four limbs. There was a short systolic murmur (3/6) heard best at the left sternal edge, radiating to the back. The femoral pulses were palpable but difficult to feel. Abdominal examination revealed a mass in each flank. His EEG is shown opposite.

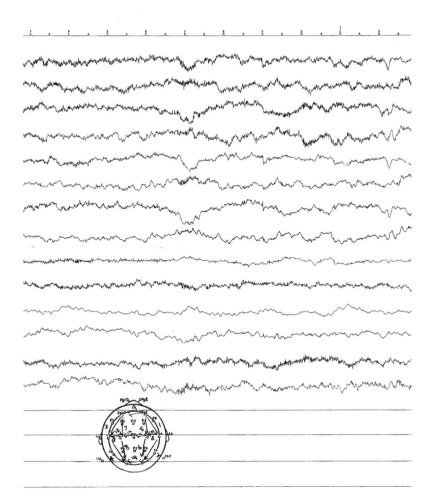

1. Give two possible causes for this infant's 'funny turn'.
2. Give three investigations you would perform.

Question 4.4

Martin can run fast and can walk up and down a flight of 12 steps, two feet to a step. He can stand on one leg for 2 seconds and stand on tiptoe. He can kick a ball forcibly and catch it with his arms extended. He is able to grip a pen in tripod fashion and can draw a circle with his left hand. He can copy a cross and build a tower of eight bricks. He says his name and knows that he is a boy, and dresses himself with some help. He washes and dries his hand when reminded.

1. How old is Martin?

Question 4.5

Over an 8-h period a 10-year-old girl developed weakness in both legs which was worst when climbing stairs. She was unable to stand within 15 h of the onset of symptoms. During this time she developed back pain and tenderness localized to the upper lumbar spine, which had become increasingly severe, and she had a temperature of 38°C. She complained of a funny feeling in her legs which felt like a 'tingling sensation'.

On examination she had loss of position and vibration sense in her feet and a reduced reaction to pin prick in the lower extremities. Muscle tone and tendon reflexes were reduced and plantar response was equivocal.

Haemoglobin	12 g/dl
White cell count	$18 \times 10^9/l$
Platelet count	$300 \times 10^9/l$
ESR	Markedly raised
Liver function tests	Normal

1. What is your clinical diagnosis?
2. Give two possible causes.
3. How may her physical signs change over the next week?

Paper 4 *ANSWERS*

Answer 4.1

1. Metabolic disorder

Sepsis

Congential heart disease

Reject: Respiratory disease
Respiratory distress syndrome

2. Serum lactate
Serum pyruvate
Plasma amino acids
Blood culture
Urine for amino acids
Urine for organic acids
Echocardiogram
Four-limb blood pressure

Serum urea and electrolytes
Full blood count
Urine culture
Septic screen

Discussion

This child has a severe metabolic acidosis which can result from a number of different causes. In this situation, these can be broadly grouped into metabolic, infective and cardiac. In the latter situation, acidosis results from hypoxia and/or hypoperfusion. There are no specific findings in this child to support such a diagnosis. Sepsis could account for this child's problems, however a presentation with profound metabolic acidosis in the absence of other blood gas abnormalities would be unusual. It would be normal practice to treat the baby with broad-spectrum antibiotics whilst cultures were awaited. A number of metabolic disorders (all rare) may result in acidosis because of the accumulation of interim products of metabolism. Several such defects, particularly those involving the urea cycle, are often accompanied by fitting. This particular child had proprionic acidaemia.

Answer 4.2

1. Hyperthyroidism
Thyrotoxicosis
Autoimmune hyperthyroidism
Graves' disease

Reject: Any answer implying secondary hyperthyroidism due to pituitary tumour or increased pituitary function

2. Carbimazole or propylthiouracil
Propranolol

Reject: Radioactive iodine
Surgery

3. Acquired hypothyroidism, secondary to treatment for hyperthyroidism

4. Thyroxine or thyroid hormone

Discussion

The early clinical history with the raised T4 and low thyroid stimulating hormone points to increased thyroid function. If pituitary hyperactivity were involved, the thyroid stimulating hormone would be high. Where thyrotoxicosis is associated with eye manifestations, Graves' disease is the more precise answer. Autonomous functioning thyroid nodules are extremely uncommon in children.

The treatment of choice in childhood is thyroid suppression by either carbimazole or propylthiouracil. Propranolol may be useful in controlling symptoms in the acute situation. The treatment of children who do not remit within 1–2 years is controversial. Although radioactive iodine and surgery are not appropriate therapy for this child, in the longer term these options are available should she not respond to medical treatment.

Following treatment for hyperthyroidism, this child has developed hypothyroidism, a recognized complication of medical treatment. The treatment is with thyroid hormone replacement.

Answer 4.3

1. Hypertensive encephalopathy
Idiopathic seizure disorder

Reject: Seizure secondary to birth asphyxia

2. Cranial ultrasound
   Abdominal ultrasound
   Echocardiogram

Discussion

The birth history suggests a degree of fetal compromise just prior to birth, but there is no evidence of postasphyxial encephalopathy in the early neonatal period, and seizures as a result of this are therefore unlikely. In view of the large head circumference compared to the other growth parameters, cranial ultrasound should be performed to exclude hydrocephalus.

The presence of bilateral flank masses suggests a renal cause for hypertension. Ultrasound scanning confirmed polycystic kidney disease. Polycystic renal disease may be inherited in either an autosomal recessive or dominant fashion. The recessive form may be associated oligohydramnios and respiratory insufficiency at birth. Renal function may be maintained into adolescence. Although the recurrence risk is 25%, there can be variable expression within siblings. The autosomal dominant form presents in adulthood in most cases, but it is occasionally seen at birth with enlarged kidneys and haematuria. Associated abnormalities include endocardial elastosis, intracerebral arteriovenous malformations, pyloric stenosis and hepatic fibrosis. As with the recessive form, variable expression is seen. Control of hypertension improves the prognosis, but renal failure eventually occurs in many survivors.

In view of the weak nature of the femoral pulses, echocardiography should be performed to exclude coarctation.

Answer 4.4

1. $2\frac{1}{2}$–3 years

Discussion

In the assessment of a child's developmental age, the categories of fine and gross motor achievements, visual and auditory development and the level of attainment of social and higher skills, e.g. speech, need to be examined. Hence, from considering each of these categories, his developmental age may be calculated.

Gross motor achievement:
$2\frac{1}{2}$ years: The child can walk up and downstairs, two feet per step. He will be able to run forward in a straight direction and kick a ball gently.
3 years: The child can walk upstairs with alternating feet and come down with two feet to each step, and can walk in any direction and kick a ball hard. Tiptoeing, standing on one leg and catching with arms extended are possible.

Fine motor achievement:
$2\frac{1}{2}$ years: Pens are held in the preferred hand with early tripod grasp and the child can draw lines and circles. A tower of 7 bricks or more can be built.

3 years: A tower of 9–12 bricks can be built. The tripod grasp is closer to the point of the pen and crosses can be drawn.

Speech:
$2\frac{1}{2}$ *years:* The child knows his name, talks whilst playing, stutters when excited and asks questions continuously.
3 years: Full name and sex said. Echolalia and continuous chatter when playing.

Social:
$2\frac{1}{2}$ *years:* Dressing is limited, being able to remove some clothes such as trousers.
3 years: Washing of hands and drying them is fine but assistance is required for zips, buttons and laces.

Answer 4.5

1. Acute paraplegia

2. Spinal epidural abscess
Post-infectious myelitis

Guillain–Barré syndrome

Syringomyelia

Reject: Hysterical paraplegia

3. Most cases will show gradual improvement, however, clear signs of paraplegia may develop:
— Definite weakness
— Definite hyper-reflexia
— Upgoing planter reflexes
— Sensory level to pin prick and/or vibration
— Loss of anal sphincter tone and absent abdominal reflexes

Discussion

In patients with acute organic paraplegia, muscle tone and tendon reflexes are often reduced in the early stages due to spinal shock. Plantar reflexes are usually, but not always, extensor and there is a change in urinary function. There is also loss of all modalities of sensation with a dermatome level corresponding to the site of the lesion. In this patient severe back pain, tenderness and fever suggest a spinal epidural abscess or a post-infectious myelitis. Some patients may present with neck stiffness suggesting subarachnoid haemorrhage from spinal angioma, meningitis secondary to spinal epidural abscess, atlantoaxial dislocation or a post-infectious myelitis.

This girl had a post-infectious myelitis. This is managed medically with dexamethasone. With treatment approximately 60% of children return to normal function and only 25% fail to show improvement. It may or may not be related to a preceding viral infection such as chickenpox or infectious mononucleosis. The cerebral spinal fluid may show a pleocytosis with increased protein and normal sugar. Myeolography is often necessary to rule out a compressive lesion.

The other likely diagnosis in this case is a spinal epidural abscess. This is a surgical emergency and is treated by laminectomy, decompression and drainage. Antibiotic therapy is given for 6 weeks to treat the underlying vertebral osteomyelitis. With prompt treatment the prognosis for full recovery is good.

Guillain–Barré syndrome is less likely in this case as back pain is so well localized and the area is tender. Other causes of spinal cord compression, which are much less likely in this case, include:

— Epidural compression (metastases, especially neuroblastoma, leukaemia and lymphoma; epidural haematoma — haemophilia and trauma; bony abnormalities — in Morquio's syndrome and trisomy 21 compression occurs at C1–C2);
— Extra-arachnoid intradural compression (neurofibroma);
— Intra-arachnoid (seeding from a cerebral tumour; dermoid cyst);
— Intramedullary compression (myoma; ependymoma; haemato- or hydromyelia).

Hysterical paraplegia is an incorrect diagnosis in this case. Features that would point to this diagnosis are:

— Contracture of antagonists during attempted movement;
— No alteration in muscle tone or reflexes;
— No retention of urine;
— A sensory loss that does not usually comply with the dermatome map and that changes during examination;
— Recent emotional upset.

Paper 5 *QUESTIONS*

Question 5.1

An infant was admitted to the neonatal unit at 3 days of age with a serum bilirubin of 480 μmol/l. He was born at 39-weeks gestation weighing 4.3 kg. Delivery was by emergency caesarian section for failure to progress. Apgar scores were 8 at 1 min and 9 at 5 min. The child had bottle fed satisfactorily. The pregnancy was largely uneventful but was closely monitored as the child's mother had undergone splenectomy 3 years earlier at the age of 25 years because of persistent thrombocytopenia. Otherwise both parents were well and this was their first child.

On examination he was not dehydrated, however he was intensely jaundiced with florid erythema toxicum. He was not bruised. There was no splenomegaly but the liver was palpable 1 cm below the costal margin in the mid-clavicular line. There were no other positive findings. The mother's blood group was AB positive and the baby's, A positive.

1. Give the most likely diagnosis?
2. Give the three most important investigations.

Question 5.2

A 3-month-old boy was admitted to hospital because of the recent development of myoclonic jerks of his limbs and head. His development was unaltered and physical examination was normal. An EEG was performed which gave the record shown overleaf:

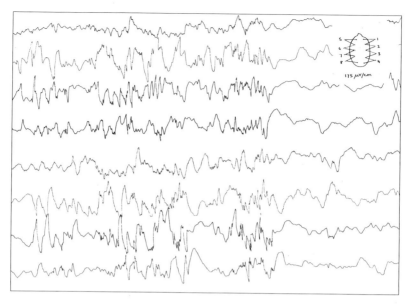

1. What is the diagnosis?
2. What two other investigations would you perform?
3. How would you treat these episodes?

Question 5.3

A 14-month-old boy was brought to casualty being given mouth-to-mouth resuscitation by his GP. The GP was called to see the child at home 1 h prior to admission with a 1-day history of fever and vomiting. Over the past few hours he had become increasingly floppy and unresponsive and shortly after the GP arrived, the child became apnoeic. He was said to have had a 'funny turn' at the age of 6 months, when he became cyanosed and unresponsive for a few seconds following a vomit. His mother was being treated for depression with tricyclic antidepressants.

Examination following intubation and ventilation revealed an appropriately grown child who was pyrexial (37.8°C). There were no external signs of injury. He made only occasional respiratory efforts, but there were no other respiratory abnormalities. His pulse was 110 beats/min, blood pressure 90/55 mmHg. There were no masses in the abdomen. His pupils were reactive but sluggish, his fundi were normal and he had a varying squint. His tone was generally reduced and his reflexes were absent apart from his plantars, which were down-going. Over the following 30 min he began to make some spontaneous movements but also had a brief generalized tonic–clonic convulsion. His pupils were noted to be unequal and he had crossed extensor reflex in his legs.

Haemoglobin	12.1 g/dl
White cell count	13.1×10^9/l
Platelet count	294×10^9/l
Sodium	128 mmol/l
Potassium	4.3 mmol/l
Urea	3.7 mmol/l
Glucose	5.1 mmol/l
Ammonia	<30 µmol/l (normal)
ECG	Sinus rhythm

1. Give three possible diagnoses.
2. What two investigations would you perform next?

Question 5.4

A 9-year-old boy presented to clinic with tall stature. On examination he was very tall, being 16 cm above the 97th centile for his age. He had arachnodactyly and his span was 7 cm greater than his height. His palate was high and arched.

On review at 10 years of age, his bone age was advanced at 12 years 6 months. On this basis his estimated final height was 2.0 m.

He had recently been referred to the ophthalmic surgeon with visual problems. The child had been referred to the paediatric clinic by a consultant cardiologist who noticed a heart murmur of aortic incompetence. Two months later he presented to hospital with acute chest pain and dyspnoea.

1. What are the two most likely underlying diagnoses?
2. How may the ophthalmologist be able to help in the differential diagnosis?
3. What two laboratory tests will help you differentiate between the most likely causes?
4. What is the cause of his dyspnoea?

Question 5.5

A 4-year-old caucasian boy presented with a week's history of bruising on his arms and legs. He was seen by his GP who referred him because of the petechial rash on his trunk. The boy had a sore throat and runny nose last week but had otherwise been well. He also complained of a severe central headache and refused to open his eyes as he said it made him see two of everything.

He was born by vaginal delivery after a normal pregnancy weighing 3.4 kg. There was no past medical history of note other than grommets being inserted at the age of 3 years. His mother was a 32-year-old housewife and his father a 34-year-old builder. They had six children: two girls aged 15 months and 6 years and three other boys aged 9, 12 and 13 years. The family lived in a four-bedroom council house in good condition. The 4-year-old boy had not been exposed to any noxious agents and had not travelled abroad.

On examination he was a pleasant boy with petechiae on the hard palate. His left eye appeared to be deviated medially. He had a soft abdomen and impalpable liver, kidneys and spleen. There were widespread petechiae, purpura and echymoses on his limbs and trunk.

Haemoglobin	11.7 g/dl
White cell count	$10.7 \times 10^9/l$
Platelet count	$30 \times 10^9/l$
Prothrombin time	16 s (control 15 s)
Partial thromboplastin time	32 s (control 31 s)
Blood group	A Rhesus positive
Atypical antibodies	None seen
Paul-Bunnell test	Negative
Blood film	Scanty platelets

1. What is the underlying condition?
2. What has occurred?
3. What three treatment steps are required immediately?

Paper 5 *ANSWERS*

Answer 5.1

1. Congenital spherocytosis
Congenital eliptocytosis

Physiological jaundice
Blood group incompatibility (not ABO)
Intrinsic red cell abnormality (e.g. G6PD deficiency or pyruvate kinase
  deficiency)
Sepsis

Reject: ABO incompatibility

2. Full blood count
Blood film
Coomb's test

Serum urea and electrolytes
Split bilirubin estimation
Liver function tests
Infection screen (LP, blood culture, urine culture)
Urine for reducing substances

Reject: Red cell fragility studies

Discussion
This baby has severe neonatal jaundice. He could have physiological jaundice, but the high bilirubin level in the absence of enhancing factors such as intrauterine growth retardation, dehydration or bruising indicate that there is likely to be an underlying cause. Sepsis may act to enhance physiological jaundice but there are no specific indications that the child is infected. Blood group incompatibility is largely excluded by the information available on the mother's and child's groups but problems can result (rarely) from incompatibilities of other red cell antigens, e.g. Duff and Kell. The mother's history of splenectomy must be considered carefully since her exact diagnosis is not given. The mother had spherocytosis which had caused splenomegaly and secondary thrombocytopenia. In reality when this mother booked for antenatal care, it was assumed her underlying diagnosis was chronic immune thrombocytopenia.

Confirmation of the diagnosis in the child, by osmotic fragility, is unreliable in the neonatal period and is normally delayed until 6 months of age.

Answer 5.2

1. Hypsarrhythmia

Reject: Epileptic focus

2. CT scans for subependymal calcification to exclude tuberose sclerosis
Skull X-ray
Renal ultrasound scan
Examination under Wood's light
Serum ammonia
CSF glycine, lactate and pyruvate
Chromosomes for trisomy 21
Mitochondrial investigation
Peroxidase investigation
Urinary amino and organic acids

3. Steroids, either prednisolone or adrenocorticotrophic hormone
Anticonvulsants, e.g. clonazepam or vigabatrin

Discussion

The EEG record shows hypsarrhythmia. There is no other interpretation for this trace and there are several known causes: tuberose sclerosis (which can be identified by calcification in the brain or hamartoma formation in the kidney), trisomy 21, mitochondrial cytopathy, peroxisomal disorders and organic acidurias. Approximately 50% of cases are idiopathic.

Although not all children will respond to therapy, steroids as either prednisolone or adrenocorticotrophic hormone have been used with some success. Other seizures may respond to anticonvulsants, in particular clonazepam or vigabatrin.

Answer 5.3

1. Meningitis
Encephalitis
Idiopathic seizure disorder

Reject: Febrile convulsion
              Tricyclic ingestion

2. Blood and throat culture
CT head scan

Reject: Lumbar puncture

Discussion

The important features in the history are the pyrexia and increasing unresponsiveness, culminating in the apnoea. These features, in addition to the physical signs, suggest intracranial sepsis as the most likely diagnosis, in this particular case being meningococcal meningitis. The main causes of death in meningitis include brain coning, massive cerebral oedema and septic shock. Any symptoms or signs suggestive of raised intracranial pressure (in this case coma, irregular respiration, unequal pupils and recent convulsive seizures) are contraindications to immediate lumbar puncture. Other clinical features suggesting raised intracranial pressure include papilloedema (although uncommon in acute meningitis), hypertension, bradycardia, absent doll's eye movements, tonic seizures, decerbrate or decorticate posture, hemiparesis and shock.

In the presence of such features, initial management should be the taking of blood and throat cultures prior to prompt instigation of intravenous antibiotic therapy and treatment for raised intracranial pressure if required. Once the child's condition is stabilized, CT should be performed to exclude conditions that may resemble meningitis with raised intracranial pressure, e.g. posterior fossa tumours, cerebral abscess, acute hydrocephalus and intracranial haemorrhage.

Answer 5.4

1. Marfan's syndrome
   Homocystinuria

2. In homocystinuria the eye lenses tend to subluxate downwards and inwards as opposed to upwards and outwards in Marfan's syndrome

3. Urine methionine
   Urine homocystine
   Urine cystine

4. Pneumothorax
   Aortic dissection
   Pulmonary embolism

Discussion

Marfan's syndrome has an incidence of 1 in 10 000 and is inherited in an autosomal dominant manner. Children with Marfan's syndrome have a tendency towards tall stature and have long slender limbs. They can have aortic incompetence, as in this child, and also may develop dilatation of the aortic root with the possibility of later dissection. Other findings include joint hyperextensibility, scoliosis, kyphosis, pectus excavatum, mitral valve prolapse, herniae (both inguinal and femoral) and myopia.

There is no characteristic facies associated with Marfan's syndrome. The lower segment of the body (symphysis pubis to heel) is longer than the upper segment. The arm span is greater than the height. Life span is shortened secondary to cardiovascular complications, particularly dissection of the aorta. Spontaneous pneumothoraxes are another common problem.

Homocystinuria has an incidence of 1 in 20 000 and is inherited in an autosomal recessive manner. The classic case will be Marfanoid in appearance. There may be connective tissue weakness producing herniae, scoliosis and cardiac complications. It differs from Marfan's syndrome in that the joints are often enlarged and stiffer rather than looser than normal. Mental retardation, strokes and heart attacks are thought to be due to vascular thromboses which may occur at any time in life, even in early infancy.

Examination of the eye lenses by an ophthalmologist may help with the differential diagnosis as they subluxate upwards and outwards in Marfan's syndrome and downwards and inwards in homocystinuria. In Marfan's syndrome other abnormalities include flat cornea, enlongated globe, retinal detachment and myopia.

The diagnosis of homocystinura may be confirmed by finding increased methionine and homocystine and decreased cystine levels in the plasma and urine.

The most likely cause of acute chest pain and dyspnoea is a pneumothorax as patients often have apical bullae which rupture. However, aortic dissection may occur and thrombotic complications in homocystinuria may lead to a pulmonary embolism.

Answer 5.5

1. Immune thrombocytopenia

Acute leukaemia

Reject: Disseminated intravascular coagulation

2. Intracranial haemorrhage

3. High doses of intravenous allogenic platelets
High dose steroids
Intravenous immunoglobulin
Urgent cranial CT
Neurosurgeon to be informed
Bone marrow examination

Discussion

The underlying condition is viral-induced immune thrombocytopenia. The previous week's history of upper respiratory tract infection, the absence of lymphadenopathy, enlarged liver or spleen make a diagnosis of myeloproliferative disorder much less likely. The normal white and red cell counts and the blood film findings support this diagnosis.

The severe central headache and the left sixth nerve palsy suggest intracranial bleeding. Urgent treatment is required as this is a life-threatening complication of immune thrombocytopenia with rates of mortality quoted as high as 50%. Only when intracranial haemorrhage complicates this condition is platelet transfusion used; high dose steroids and immunoglobin are given to raise the endogenous platelet count.

Cranial CT will localize the site of bleeding and close observation will be required as deterioration may require craniotomy; hence the neurosurgeon must be informed as soon as the condition is suspected.

Bone marrow examination may score some marks if the candidate is considering that the cranial nerve disorder and headache are components of a presentation of acute leukaemia with cranial involvement.

Paper 6 *QUESTIONS*

Question 6.1

A 4-week-old baby was brought to clinic with feeding problems. She was born at 38-weeks gestation weighing 3.5 kg. The baby required intubation at birth but was extubated by 15 min of age. The baby then spent 3 days in the neonatal unit with irritability and poor feeding. She continued to make slow progress and eventually left hospital with her mother when she was 8 days old.

After discharge she became increasingly difficult to feed. When offered a bottle, she often struggled and arched and rarely took more than 60–90 ml at a time. She vomited infrequently and her stools were not loose or watery. Between feeds the baby tended to be irritable and slept very little.

The baby was difficult to examine since she cried when disturbed. Her weight was 3.7 kg. Tone appeared generally increased and tendon reflexes were brisk. A feed was observed: the child struggled but eventually took 90 ml and did not vomit afterwards.

1. What is the diagnosis?
2. Suggest the most important investigation.

Question 6.2

A 12-year-old girl with haemoglobin SS disease presented with bilateral anterior chest pains, which were worse with inspiration and associated with dyspnoea. She had had a fever and symptoms of an upper respiratory tract infection over the past week. She had regularly taken penicillin and in the past had had frequent admissions to hospital with joint and limb pains, but she had not experienced similar chest symptoms before.

On examination her respiratory rate was 28 breaths/min with bilateral vesicular breath sounds. There was slight tenderness over T4 to L1 vertebral bodies but there were no other abnormal physical signs. Her temperature was 37.6°C.

Haemoglobin	7.3 g/dl
White cell count	$17.8 \times 10^9/l$
Lymphocytes	80%
Neutrophils	15%
Platelet count	$289 \times 10^9/l$
Urea and electrolytes	Normal
Serum bilirubin	44 mmol/l
Protein	83 g/dl
Alanine transferase	33 IU/l

Alkaline phosphatase	165 IU/l
Chest X-ray	Normal
Oxygen saturation in air	88%

1. What is the diagnosis?
2. Give the two most important treatment steps?
3. How does this episode alter the long-term management of this patient?

Question 6.3

A 6-year-old girl presented to hospital with left-sided weakness of acute onset. There had been no associated recent ill health and no history of headache, vomiting, visual disturbance or trauma. In the past year, however, there had been some concern over possible increasing clumsiness and she was thought to be rather slow with her school work. She had always been left handed. She had three older siblings, all of whom were well. Both paternal grandparents died in their early 50s from myocardial infarction, and a maternal aunt had a haemorrhagic stroke at the age of 49 years.

The main findings on examination were an alert, well orientated child with normal blood pressure, normal cardiovascular system and a dense left hemiparesis with an upgoing plantar reflex on the left side. There were no neurocutaneous stigmata. Over the next 12 h her hemiparesis resolved. Investigations including full blood count, clotting screen, metabolic screen, lipoprotein profile and echocardiogram were all normal and there was no evidence of infection. A CT head scan showed a small area of periventricular white matter infarction on the left side, which did not appear acute.

She was discharged home but readmitted 4 weeks later with a further episode of left-sided weakness. She also complained of tingling in the right arm and leg and was noted to be dysphasic. She remained normotensive and there were no other new findings. A repeat CT scan showed bilateral areas of infarction of both hemispheres.

1. What investigation would you consider performing next?
2. Suggest a diagnosis.

Question 6.4

A 5-week-old infant presented with a history of persistent vomiting, poor feeding and pyrexia. His conscious state was markedly depressed. Initial blood results showed a pH of 7.0 and $PaCO_2$ of 3.5 kPa. Blood glucose was 1.5 mmol/l and liver function tests were mildly abnormal. Following correction of the acidosis and hypoglycaemia, intravenous antibiotics and ventilation for a subsequent apnoeic episode, the infant recovered. Lumbar puncture was normal and there was no growth from blood cultures or suprapubic aspiration of urine. Serum protein was normal. The possibility of a metabolic abnormality was raised.

1. What four factors in this case history point towards the diagnosis of a metabolic disease?
2. Give four important questions to ask in taking a history when a metabolic disease is suspected.
3. Give four further tests which need to be performed when a metabolic disease is suspected.

Question 6.5

You are called to the labour ward to attend in the resuscitation of a full-term baby who has fetal distress. The delivery is vaginal and the baby only requires face-mask oxygen and nasopharyngeal suction. The Apgar score at 1 min is 9 and at 5 min 10.

The midwife informs you that the mother has been in contact with hepatitis B, and at the time of birth she is positive to the hepatitis B surface antigen, negative to the e antigen and has antibodies to the e component.

1. What, if any, treatment does the baby need?

Paper 6 *ANSWERS*

Answer 6.1

1. Post-asphyxial cerebral damage

Reflux oesophagitis
Infantile colic

Occult infection, e.g. urinary tract infection
Neurodegenerative disorder

Reject: Pyloric stenosis
Food allergy

2. Cranial CT scan
Cranial ultrasound scan
MRI scan

Barium meal
pH probe
EEG

Urine culture
Investigations relevant to cerebral degenerative disease

Discussion

This child has suffered a significant perinatal insult resulting in considerable cerebral damage. The condition at birth does not always reflect the severity of the insult that has occurred and indeed may be normal. Feeding difficulties sometimes accompanied by fits and/or irritable behaviour are commonly found in this group of babies and may antedate other clear evidence of neurological damage. The history is sufficient to suggest this diagnosis but the other conditions listed all merit consideration, particularly gastro-oesophageal reflux.

Cranial imaging (by whatever means) at 6 weeks following the insult will commonly demonstrate considerable cerebral atrophy and therefore support the diagnosis. Of the three investigations given, MRI is probably the most sensitive in this situation but is not readily available.

Answer 6.2

1. Acute sickle cell chest syndrome
   Atypical chest infection

   Sickle cell crisis
   Chest infection or pneumonia

2. Oxygen
   Exchange transfusion

   Simple blood transfusion
   Antibiotics

   Pain relief

3. Regular blood transfusion regimen

Discussion

The acute chest syndrome is a particularly sinister development in sickle cell disease and is one of the commonest causes of death in this illness. It is characterized by increasing dyspnoea and is probably a combination of both infection and infarction. Sickle signs may be unimpressive and a chest X-ray may appear normal initially. Any answer that does not include the possibility of infection or infarction is incorrect. A simple chest infection is possible, although it is unlikely to be bilateral without underlying sickling, and as such is only a partly correct answer.

The treatment involves oxygen and an exchange transfusion to decrease the percentage of sickle cells below 20. This may require several exchange transfusions. Antibiotics are also important and some consideration should be given to an atypical bacterial infection. Pain relief is important but as an answer earns fewer marks than the others.

The long-term management of patients who have had the acute chest syndrome remains controversial. Many authorities recommend a regular blood transfusion regimen over the subsequent few months in order to allow resolution of the infarction. Should this condition recur, then a long-term programme of transfusions should be instituted. This would of course require iron chelation therapy as an adjunct.

Answer 6.3

1. Cerebral angiography

2. Vascular malformation
   Vascular occlusive disease
   Moyamoya disease

Discussion

Causes of acute hemiplegia may be broadly divided into vascular malformations (arteriovenous malformations, aneurysms and microangiomas), arterial occlusive disease (arteritis, vasospasm, hypertension, spontaneous arterial occlusion), venous occlusion (thrombosis), cerebral disease (peri-ictal, encephalitis, abscess, tumours, multiple sclerosis), subdural haematomas and migraine. The presentation of this girl suggests widespread arterial occlusion as a likely cause, due in this case to Moyamoya disease, although a vascular malformation is a more likely cause. Moyamoya disease is a progressive, bilateral cerebral arterial disease. It is sporadic with no predisposing factors. About half of the cases present before 10 years of age and 70% before 20 years, commonly with acute hemiplegia, transient dysphagia or other acute deficits with and without seizures. Recurrent transient ischaemic attacks are an alternative manifestation, characterized by episodic hemiparesis and dysesthesias lasting minutes to hours.

Answer 6.4

1. Persistent vomiting
Poor feeding
Depressed conscious state and apnoea
Deranged liver function
Acidosis
Hypoglycaemia

2. Is there a family history of neonatal death or consanguinity?
Was the baby normal for a period after birth?
What type of feeding was given initially?
Has there been a change in feeding with respect to the protein, sugar or fat content?
Has anything occurred to the baby which might precipitate metabolic disease, e.g. infection, prolonged fasting or surgery?
Has the baby improved on intravenous glucose, fluids, and relapsed after recommencement of milk feeds?

3. Simple spot test for urinary pH, ketones, ketoacids and non-glucose reducing substances
Blood glucose, blood gases, serum electrolytes, calcium, magnesium, liver function tests and full blood count
Amino acid profile on blood and urine
Urine for organic acids
Screening test for galactosaemia
Plasma ammonia
Plasma ketone bodies

Discussion

Diagnosis of an inborn error of metabolism is important for a number of reasons. In childhood it may lead to specific treatment and increased chance of survival. The earlier the diagnosis is made, the greater the chance that children capable of survival will do so without neurological sequelae and that the lives of infants with lethal diseases will not be prolonged unnecessarily. For parents and relatives, diagnosis leads to accurate genetic counselling. Diagnosis needs to be established during life, since post-morten diagnosis is usually impossible unless substantial progress towards a diagnosis has been made before death.

Treatment of children with metabolic diseases depends on the precise defect present. However, some general principles of treatment exist. The major component of the treatment of a sick newborn is general supportive care, including correction of hypoglycaemia, acidosis and hypotension, exchange transfusion for marked jaundice or acidosis, antibiotics, anticonvulsants, ventilation and correction of clotting abnormalities.

Feeds should cease and intravenous glucose commenced. This has the effect of removing those components of food that cannot be metabolized, e.g. galactose in galactosaemia. However, some forms of lactic acidosis may be aggravated by a high carbohydrate intake. In some cases toxic metabolites may be removed by exchange transfusion or peritoneal dialysis.

Answer 6.5

1. Vaccination and hepatitis immunoglobulin are both required

Discussion

Although vertical transmission is most likely when the maternal serology is hepatitis B e antigen positive, cases of transmission have been reported from mothers who have antibody to e antigen. In this latter group, viral replication can still occur and even if antibody has been elaborated, the baby could still be at risk. Hence the current recommendations are that both passive and active immunization should be given, i.e. the first dose of vaccine should be given preferably within the first 12 h of life, 0.5 ml (10 µg) intramuscularly into the anterolateral aspect of the thigh (in preference to the deltoid). The hepatitis immunoglobulin (200 IU) should be given into the contralateral thigh by intramuscular injection. Repeated doses of vaccine should be given at 1 month and at 6 months of age. Seroconversion should be checked when the child is 1 year.

Paper 7 *QUESTIONS*

Question 7.1

A 4-year-old girl was brought to casualty. Whilst helping her to get dressed that morning her mother noticed some bruising of the child's labia majora. She could not recall her daughter falling or injuring herself in any way. Otherwise the child was completely well and had never had any significant medical problems.

In the family there were two older sisters aged 6 and 8 years, both of whom were well. Both parents were in good health but they had separated 12 months earlier. The three girls now lived with their mother and her partner.

On examination the child was cooperative, clean and well dressed. She had grown normally and had no bruises on her limbs. General examination was normal. Examination of the genitalia revealed some minor abrasions to the labia majora but the labia minora and the vaginal orifice appeared normal. The anus and surrounding skin were reddened, however the anus was not dilated.

1. What is the diagnosis?
2. What would be the next step in this child's management?

Question 7.2

A 7-month-old girl was admitted with a 5-day history of an upper respiratory tract infection. Diarrhoea had developed over the last 2 days. There was no blood or mucus. Her appetite was poor. She was treated before presentation to hospital with cotrimoxazole and a balanced electrolyte solution. On the morning of admission she was found by her parents, staring, unresponsive, floppy, tachypnoeic and with a dry nappy, not having drunk since going to bed 12 h before. She had had one brief staring episode in the past but otherwise her previous medical history and development had been normal. A sister died of a cot death 2 years previously and there were no other siblings. Both parents were well.

On examination her temperature was 35.7°C, pulse 140 beats/min, blood pressure 105/45 mmHg and there were scattered crepitations throughout her lungs. She was generally hypotonic but there was no asymmetry. Her Glasgow coma score was 12. The remainder of the examination was normal. In the A&E department, her blood sugar was 1 mmol/l and she was treated with intravenous dextrose. Over the next 12 h her blood sugar increased and she improved and was alert. She was treated with intravenous acyclovir and antibiotics and the next day a lumbar puncture was performed which was normal.

Investigations on admission

Haemoglobin	11.1 g/dl
White cell count	14.5×10^9/l
Platelet count	530×10^9/l
Urea and electrolytes	Normal
Creatinine	29 mmol/l
pH	7.3
$PaCO_2$	5 kPa
Bicarbonate	17 mmol/l
Base excess	−8.8 mmol/l
Calcium	2.46 mmol/l
Magnesium	0.96 mmol/l
Ammonia	18 μmol/l (normal <40 μmol/l)
Pyruvate	50 mg/l (normal 40–138 mg/l)
Lactate	0.8 mmol/l (normal 0.5–1.8 mmol/l)
INR	1.2
Liver function tests	Normal
Urinary reducing substances	Negative
Ketones	Negative
CSF glycine	Normal
Rotavirus	Isolated in stools

1. What is the likely diagnosis?
2. What two investigations would confirm this?

Question 7.3

A 3-year-old boy was brought to casualty following a generalized convulsion. He had been well until 4 days prior to admission, when he had developed malaise, vomiting and a pyrexia which had not responded to paracetamol. In the past he had pneumonia associated with measles and was circumcised 6 months previously for difficulty in micturition. A first cousin had Duchenne muscular dystrophy.

Whilst being assessed he had a further generalized convulsion, which required several anticonvulsants to control. His perfusion and respiratory effort were noted to be poor and he was therefore intubated and transferred to the intensive care unit. On examination he was pyrexial (39°C), with a macular rash on his trunk. There were a few petechiae on his chest. There was a mass palpable in both flanks. His optic disc margins were blurred, his tone was increased in his legs compared to his arms and his reflexes were generally brisk with marked ankle clonus.

Haemoglobin	10.2 g/dl
White cell count	15.2×10^9/l
Platelet count	61×10^9/l
INR	1.6

1. What is the most likely diagnosis?
2. What is the underlying abnormality?
3. What further history would you try to elicit?
4. What two investigations would you perform next?

Question 7.4

An 18-month-old child was referred to the paediatric surgical team following drainage of a large staphylococcal abscess on his right thigh. History revealed he had suffered from recurrent small boils and had had three episodes of impetigo which seemed to spread from his nose. He had suffered two previous abscesses on his buttocks but these responded to high-dose flucloxacillin. There was no evidence of eczema or any other skin lesions, and on examination there were no abnormal findings. His 5-year-old brother also had a history of less severe but recurrent boils to the legs, buttocks and neck. These were treated with flucloxacillin with good results.

Haemoglobin	13 g/dl
MCV	80 fl
White cell count	13×10^9/l
Blood glucose	4.3 mmol/l
Liver function tests	Normal
Urea and electrolytes and creatinine	Normal
Blood culture	No growth
Culture from abscess drained surgically	*Staphylococcus aureus*

1. Give three further investigations you would perform.
2. How would you treat recurrent staphylococcal skin infections, assuming no abnormalities were found on further investigation?

Question 7.5

A 2-year-old boy was referred as he was having episodes of becoming dusky. These episodes had been increasing in frequency over the past 3 months. They lasted initially for a few minutes but now lasted 5–10 min. They did not occur more often with exercise.

He was born at full term by vaginal delivery and had been otherwise well. He was up to date with immunizations and had achieved his developmental milestones appropriately. His father was a 38-year-old biochemist and his mother a 34-year-old head teacher of a comprehensive school. There was no family history of note.

On examination he was clubbed and appeared to be centrally cyanosed. He was not anaemic but appeared lethargic. More detailed cardiorespiratory findings were:

Pulse rate	80 beats/min
Cardiac palpation	Parasternal heave on left lower sternal border, systolic thrill over lower and middle left sternal border
First heart sound	Normal
Second heart sound	Only aortic component heard
Respiratory rate	40 breaths/min
Chest	Clear

The following ECG was taken:

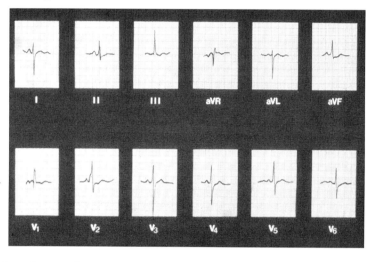

1. What abnormalities are present from the ECG?

This was his chest X-ray:

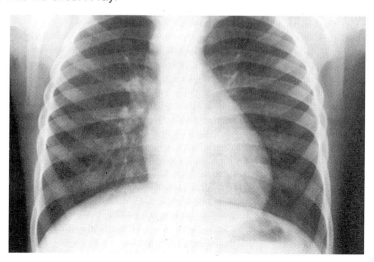

2. What abnormalities are present from the chest X-ray?

Suddenly he became increasingly tachypnoeic and more cyanosed. He became limp and slumped to the floor. His murmur was no longer audible.

3. What is happening?
4. What three things should be done?

Paper 7 *ANSWERS*

Answer 7.1

1. Thread worms

Local irritation, e.g. allergic to washing powder
Masturbation
Lichen planus

Reject: Non-accidental injury
Sexual abuse

2. Test for thread worms, e.g. cellotape test

Ask for senior medical advice

Reject: Take place of safety order
Take emergency protection order
Contact social services
Call case conference
Contact police
Skeletal survey
Clotting studies
Take clinical photographs

Discussion

This child has thread worms and has been scratching in her sleep. It could be argued in view of the history that the initial examination should have been by a senior paediatrician and a police surgeon. Similarly, it would have been normal practice to consult the 'at risk' register prior to seeing such a child. However, the evidence on examination is clearly of superficial irritation with no suggestion of anything more sinister. The cellotape test confirms the presence of thread worms.

Answer 7.2

1. Medium chain acyl CoA dehydrogenase deficiency
Fatty acid oxidation defect

Reject: Reye's syndrome
Leigh's encephalopathy
Galactosaemia

      Encephalitis
      Meningitis
      Urea cycle defect
      Haemorrhagic shock
      Haemolytic uraemic syndrome
      Non-ketotic hypoglycaemia

2. Urinary amino and organic acid screen
    L-carnitine load

Discussion

This child presents with an acute encephalopathy for which there are a number of causes, but the information given excludes a number of conditions as above. Particular features of this child are the hypoglycaemia and the death of a sibling with sudden infant death syndrome (SIDS). Medium chain acyl CoA dehydrogenase deficiency is a well-recognized cause of SIDS. Her response to intravenous glucose and her previous staring episode, which suggests a recurring problem, also support the diagnosis. This child has had an acute infection, i.e. rotavirus, which has provoked hypoglycaemia because of her enzyme deficiency.

The diagnosis is confirmed by a characteristic increase in urinary organic acids. An L-carnitine load also produces an increase in octanoylcarnitine.

Answer 7.3

1. Septicaemia with evidence of consumptive coagulopathy
2. Urinary tract infection secondary to obstructive uropathy
3. Evidence of poor urinary stream
4. Urine microscopy and culture
    Abdominal ultrasound

Discussion

This boy has posterior urethral valves as the underlying cause of his illness as suggested by palpable renal masses. In boys presenting with difficulty in micturition it is important to obtain information regarding urinary stream. Urine microscopy and culture is important to confirm the source of infection and abdominal ultrasound will reveal hydronephrosis, hydroureter and a trabeculated bladder wall. Management will be directed at treating the septicaemia and relieving renal obstruction acutely before definitive treatment for urethral valves.

Answer 7.4

1. Leucocyte differential count
Albumin/globulin ratio
Immunoglobulins G, A, M and E and antibody titres
Complement C3, C4 and CH50
Neutrophil function tests

2. Flucloxacillin
Anti-staphylococcal measures:
— non-sensitizing chlorhexidine compounds reduce the likelihood of re-infection
— nasal chlorhexidine cream
— Cidal soap

Discussion

The leucocyte and differential counts will give absolute numbers of neutrophils and monocytes. If infections are occurring regularly, then weekly differential counts should be performed to exclude cyclical neutropenia. Neutrophil function defects are often associated with neutrophilia and hyper-gammaglobulinaemia. An albumin:globulin ratio should be about 1.5. A raised globulin, and therefore a low ratio, may be an appropriate response to recurrent infection but may alternatively be an attempt to compensate for neutrophil or antibody deficiency.

Immunoglobulin and IgM antibody titres and complement levels confirm humoral adequacy. If IgE levels are absolutely quantitated and are normal then the hyper-IgE syndrome will be excluded.

The screening neutrophil function test is the NBT — a simple assay of the respiratory burst — and is an essential part of the investigation of these children. Bacterial killing assays should also be performed. If bacterial killing is abnormal but the NBT test is normal, defects of chemotaxis, opsinization and adherence should be sought.

Treatment with flucloxacillin may be useful, but should be given in conjunction with the topical measures mentioned above. If the staphylococcal infection recurs, cultures from the family may identify the carrier and all household members should receive the above regimen. Topical pseudomonic acid may be effective at clearing nasal carriage.

Answer 7.5

1. Right axis deviation ($+120° - +150°$)
Right ventricular hypertrophy
Right atrial hypertrophy

2. Oligaemia
Concave mediastinal shadow in the region of the main pulmonary artery
Right atrial enlargement
Right-sided aortic arch

Reject: Cardiac arrhythmia
            Methaemoglobinaemia

3. Fallot's tetralogy in acute 'spell'

4. a) Place in the knee–chest position to increase the systemic vascular resistance
   b) Intravenous administration of morphine to help with central sedation
   c) Intravenous administration of propranolol to reduce the pulmonary infundibular spasm
   d) Treat acidosis, e.g. with colloid/crystalloid or bicarbonate
   e) If persistent or severe, an intravenous infusion of noradrenaline should be commenced to increase the systemic vascular resistance
   f) Oxygen therapy will not immediately alleviate the pulmonary infudibular spasm, however it is often given to ameliorate cyanosis

Discussion

His ECG and chest X-ray are consistent with tetralogy of Fallot and the clinical presentation of becoming limp and cyanosed with loss of murmur is classic of a 'spell'. In a cyanotic spell there is acute right ventricular outflow tract obstruction with reversal of blood across the ventricular septal defect.

Cardiac arrhythmia would not fit with the ECG and chest X-ray findings. Methaemoglobinaemia would not have an episodic presentation as the cyanosis would be present continuously.

Paper 8 *QUESTIONS*

Question 8.1

A 7-year-old boy was referred with nocturnal enuresis. He had consistently wet at night throughout his life. He was otherwise a normal, happy child. He had two older sisters who were both well and both had been dry day and night since 4 years of age. His mother was well but as a child had wet the bed until 10 years of age. His father suffered from insulin-dependent diabetes mellitus. At the time of referral both parents were out of work.

In order to try and control the problem, the child's fluid intake during the evening had been reduced. However, the family had tried no other measures.

On examination he was cooperative and well grown; his weight was on the 50th centile and height on the 75th. There were no abnormal findings.

1. What would be your initial approach to management?
2. Give the most important investigation.

Question 8.2

A 3-year-old boy was referred to hospital by his GP with severe epistaxis and multiple bruising on his limbs. He had previously been well and there were no other abnormalities on physical examination. He had not had any drugs. The family was well.

Haemoglobin	10.3 g/dl
White cell count	$13.3 \times 10^9/l$
Neutrophils	43%
Lymphocytes	30%
Platelet count	$3 \times 10^9/l$
INR	1.3
Urea and electrolytes	Normal
Liver function tests	Normal
Platelet antibodies	Negative
ESR	20 mm/h

1. What is the likely diagnosis?
2. What single investigation would you perform and why?
3. What is the treatment?

Question 8.3

A 1-day-old male infant was referred for investigation for cyanosis. He was born at term, birthweight 3.5 kg, being the second child of healthy unrelated parents. Pregnancy and delivery had been uneventful. Central cyanosis was noted after delivery, with no apparent respiratory distress. Pulses were normal and a soft systolic murmur was heard at the left sternal edge. His brother had pyloric stenosis as an infant, requiring pyloromyotomy.

At the time of transfer he was noted to be extremely cyanosed (oxygen saturation 42%) and had a marked metabolic acidosis. Echocardiography revealed transposition of the great arteries and an emergency balloon septostomy was performed, with immediate improvement in oxygen saturation and acid–base status. After a further 24 h he developed abdominal distension with bile-stained vomiting. On examination he looked unwell with poor peripheral perfusion. Cardiovascular examination was unchanged. The abdomen was distended and difficult to palpate.

The abdominal X-ray was:

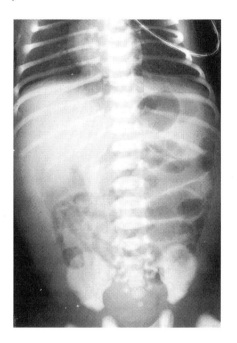

Haemoglobin	15.7 g/dl
White cell count	$12.5 \times 10^9/l$
Platelet count	$210 \times 10^9/l$
Sodium	133 mmol/l
Potassium	4.3 mmol/l
Urea	5.1 mmol/l
Glucose	4.1 mmol/l

1. What is the most likely diagnosis?
2. What abnormality is seen on the X-ray?
3. How should the case be managed?

Question 8.4

A 22-year-old woman presented in established labour at term. She had had a normal pregnancy and was well apart from the appearance 24 h before labour commenced of a mild pustular rash. There was no history of previous skin complaints although there had been an outbreak of chickenpox in her neighbourhood.

A healthy boy was delivered and both mother and child were discharged from hospital 3 days later. Twelve h later, the mother represented with her son who had developed a severe pustular rash.

1. What is the most likely diagnosis?
2. How would you manage this child?
3. If you had seen the child following delivery, what would you have done?

Question 8.5

A 12-year-old boy was brought to casualty by his parents. He had been difficult to rouse that morning from sleep and had been slurring his speech the previous day. He had not vomited but felt nauseous. He complained of central headache radiating to the back of his head, a dull consistent pain not relieved by simple analgesia. This headache had started that morning and slowly became worse.

He was a second twin born at 34-weeks gestation and had since been otherwise well. He had not had any recent illnesses. He had had measles at 14 months and chickenpox at 6 years. He was fully immunized and had had BCG. There was no history of drug ingestion or drug abuse. He had been making satisfactory progress at school. His mother was a 32-year-old housewife and his father a 34-year-old sales assistant. His parents and twin sister were well.

On examination he appeared confused but answered to direct questions and was orientated in time and space. His oral temperature was 37.5°C. His Glasgow coma score was 15. In the cardiovascular system his pulse was 60 beats/min and regular. His blood pressure in the right arm was 120/70 mmHg. Heart sounds included normal first and second heard without additional sounds. The respiratory examination revealed a respiratory rate of 15 breaths/min and no distress. His chest was clear on auscultation and normal to percussion. Abdominal examination was unremarkable. Within the central nervous system, cranial nerves were intact and pupils equal and reactive.

Fundoscopy showed normal discs and no venous/arterial abnormality. Tendon reflexes, power and tone in limbs and trunk were normal. Plantar reflexes were downgoing on testing. He had neck stiffness and positive Kernig's sign.

Haemoglobin	14.7 g/dl
White cells count	20×10^9/l
Platelet count	394×10^9/l
Serum sodium	139 mmol/l
Serum potassium	3.8 mmol/l
Serum urea	5.4 mmol/l
Serum creatine	47 mmol/l
Serum glucose	8.3 mmol/l
Total bilirubin	4 mmol/l
Total protein	82 g/dl
Albumin	42 g/dl
Alanine transferase	14 µmol/l
Ammonia	17 µmol/l (normal <40 µmol/l)

Blood cultures, serum vital titres and serum and urine toxicology screen were taken.

1. What is this clinical picture?
2. What treatment should be started?

Paper 8 ANSWERS

Answer 8.1

1. Star chart (or variant)
   Bell and pad system
   Intranasal DDAVP
   Bladder control training programme
   Oxybutinin

Reject: Referral to child psychiatrist

2. Urine culture and microscopy
   Urine osmolarity and urea and electrolytes

   Urine stick test for blood, protein and sugar

Reject: Abdominal ultrasound scan
   Intravenous pyelogram
   Renal isotope scan

Discussion

This child has a primary enuresis with a good supporting family history. There is nothing to suggest an underlying disorder and any investigation at this stage should be limited.

A simple reward system (star chart) is probably the best approach. Alarm systems are sometimes frightening but they will work for some children. Intranasal DDAVP will usually produce a temporary relief of symptoms, and oxybutinin is effective, too.

Answer 8.2

1. Acute idiopathic thrombocytopenic purpura
   Post-infectious thrombocytopenia
   Acute leukaemia

Reject: Disseminated intravascular coagulopathy
   Drug-induced thrombocytopenia
   Autoimmune disease
   Haemolytic uraemic syndrome

2. Bone marrow aspiration to exclude leukaemia

  3. Expectant
     Prednisolone
     Intravenous pooled immunoglobulin

Discussion

This is a common presentation in paediatric practice. The differential diagnosis always includes acute leukaemia. Pointers which do not support acute leukaemia include his normal haemoglobin and the differential white cell count. Nevertheless, it remains a possibility despite these findings. The ESR is not consistent with autoimmune disease and the normal urea and electrolytes exclude haemolytic uraemic syndrome. The normal clotting excludes disseminated intravascular coagulopathy.

The important investigation is a bone marrow aspiration, particularly if steroid therapy is planned. The need for this aspiration is controversial and many centres do not consider this necessary unless there is any doubt about the diagnosis.

Similarly, treatment for idiopathic thrombocytopenia is controversial. Although prednisolone and intravenous pooled immunoglobin have been recommended and there is some evidence that their use has shortened the period of thrombocytopenia in the acute phase, there is no evidence that this improves the long-term outcome. Because of this some units choose not to start treatment unless there is evidence of active bleeding.

Answer 8.3

1. Necrotizing enterocolitis
   Bowel ischaemia
   Small bowel atresia
   Volvulus

Reject: Pyloric stenosis

2. Gaseous distension
   Free air in pentaneal cavity

3. Conservative if no perforation
   Surgical repair and/or bowel resection if perforation has occurred

Discussion

This child has several factors which might predispose to necrotizing enterocolitis (hypoxia and acidosis prior to septostomy). In addition, balloon septostomy has also been associated with subsequent development of this condition. The reasons for this are uncertain, but suggestions include interference with bowel venous drainage by the septostomy catheter and as a result of the venous pressure wave caused during septostomy.

Answer 8.4

1. Neonatal chickenpox
2. Admission and treatment with intravenous acyclovir
3. Zoster immune globulin is recommended, following delivery, for infants of women who develop chickenpox within a few days of (before or after) delivery. Parents are asked to return with their child as soon as the chickenpox rash is noted, and are then treated with acyclovir

Discussion

Maternal infection in late pregnancy is associated with perinatal infection in 20–60% of cases. A rash may be present at birth or develop in a few days. If the onset of maternal infection occurs between about 5 days before and 2 days after delivery, the chickenpox may be severe with a relatively short incubation period (mean 11 days) and onset at 5–10 days of age. Chickenpox occurring before this time usually results in a mild neonatal infection. A neonatal mortality of 20–30% has been recorded when the onset is between 5 days before and 2 days after delivery of the infected mother.

Pregnant women who are believed to be susceptible (on the basis of history and preferably assay of serum antibodies) and have exposure to chickenpox, should be given zoster immune globulin. Although this can prevent or modify clinical varicella, there is no evidence that it prevents fetal damage or infection.

Zoster immune globulin is also recommended for infants of women who develop chickenpox within a few days of delivery (before or after). Severe neonatal infection should be treated with intravenous acyclovir which is safe and can improve the outcome appreciably.

Answer 8.5

1. Acute meninigo-encephalopathy
   Drug/solvent abuse

Reject: Munchausen by proxy

2. Fluid restriction
   Acyclovir 500 mg/m^2 t.i.d. for a minimum of 10 days
   Broad-spectrum antibiotics given intravenously whilst awaiting culture results
   Dexamethasone before administration of antibiotics

Discussion

Children who have acute encephalopathy usually present with a short history of altered consciousness accompanied by focal neurological signs and seizures. The signs in this case are of meningism with a confused state, indicating an encephalopathic element but drug and solvent abuse have not been excluded.

As bacterial and viral meningitis may present in this fashion, treatment must be started against any possible agents. Fluid restriction is used to reduce cerebral oedema and to counteract inappropriate antidiuretic hormone production which may arise. Antibiotics with broad cover and good cerebrospinal fluid penetration should be used. Dexamethasone is used to reduce the incidence or neurological sequelae subsequent to bacterial meningitis. If there is an encephalitic element, acyclovir must be started. Serum herpes titres are of little value in this diagnosis.

Paper 9 QUESTIONS

Question 9.1

An 18-month-old boy was brought to clinic because he had not yet started to walk. He was born at 32-weeks gestation as a vertex delivery following spontaneous premature labour. Apgar scores had been 6 at 1 min and 9 at 5 min. The baby had developed mild idiopathic respiratory distress syndrome and required head box oxygen for about 48 h. He had subsequently done well and was discharged at 3 weeks of age, fully breast fed. Following discharge he had made good progress. He first smiled at 14 weeks after birth, was grasping and mouthing objects by 6 months and could crawl vigourously by 9 months.

He was the second child in the family. A girl born 4 years previously died as a cot death at the age of 4 months. Both parents were nurses and enjoyed good health.

On examination the boy was normally grown. Muscle power was normal but tone was a little reduced. He was observed to pull to stand for a few seconds but he made no attempt to walk. The remainder of the examination was normal.

1. What is the diagnosis?
2. Give the most important investigation.

Question 9.2

A 3-month-old baby was brought urgently to the A&E department after becoming blue and apnoeic whilst feeding. The episode lasted about 30 s and the baby started breathing after stimulation by the parents. Physical examination was entirely normal and the baby had had no other symptoms in the past. During admission a chest X-ray and oesophageal pH monitoring study were performed and the results are shown overleaf.

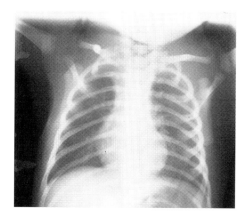

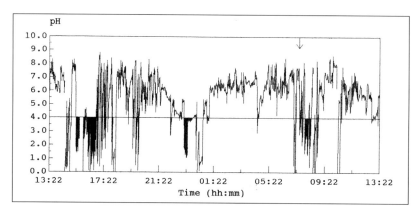

1. What is the diagnosis?

Question 9.3

A boy was born at term weighing 3.4 kg and was the first child of healthy parents. The mother's blood group was B Rhesus positive. Delivery was complicated by meconium aspiration, and the baby required oxygen via a hood (maximum FiO_2 0.65) for the first 24 h of life. An umbilical arterial catheter was inserted to monitor blood gases during this time, but was removed once supplemental oxygen was discontinued. Subsequently the infant developed necrotizing enterocolitis with perforation the following day, necessitating laparotomy. At operation, extensive changes compatible with necrotizing enterocolitis were found in the large bowel, but it was felt that resection was not required. The perforation was oversewn and a defunctioning ileostomy formed.

The infant remained unstable in the postoperative period, needing ventilatory support. He received large volumes of both blood and colloid to maintain adequate circulatory volume and also required platelet transfusion. Because of the large transfusion requirements, some O Rhesus negative red cell concentrates and platelets were used (the infant's blood group was B Rhesus negative). Over the following 24 h, large amounts of colloid support continued to be required to maintain blood pressure, and he became oedematous and increasingly difficult to ventilate. In addition, he remained relatively anaemic despite repeated transfusion and he passed frankly blood-stained urine. He was noted to be deeply jaundiced and subsequently required several exchange transfusions.

Haemoglobin	11.3 g/dl
White cell count	$3.7 \times 10^9/l$
Platelet count	$113 \times 10^9/l$
Direct Coomb's test	Weakly positive (IgG)
Blood film	Red cell agglutination, some spherocytes
Urine microscopy	No red cells, 10 white cells, scanty granular casts
INR	1.4
Total bilirubin (post exchange)	275 µmol/l, 26 µmol/l direct

1. Give three possible causes for this infant's hyperbilirubinaemia.
2. How would you manage the child's subsequent course?

Question 9.4

A 6-month-old child was referred for assessment of a respiratory problem. Symptoms developed insidiously at about 9 weeks of age with a variable inspiratory and expiratory stridor. Over the last month the severity of the stridor had increased, and the child had developed a croupy cough but had a normal cry. There had been no weight gain over the last 3 weeks. His respiratory difficulty became much worse when he cried or struggled.

The parents had been told that the most likely diagnosis was that of an infantile larynx. His chest X-ray was normal and a follow-up appointment was made for 6 weeks later.

1. What information in the case history makes the diagnosis of infantile larynx unlikely?
2. What are the two most likely diagnoses?
3. Which two further investigations do you consider most important to request next in this case?

Question 9.5

A 7-week-old girl was brought to casualty with a history of poor feeding. Her mother, a 39-year-old chief electrician, gave birth in another local casualty department by spontaneous vaginal delivery at 36-weeks gestation. The girl's birthweight was 2.1 kg and the occipitofrontal circumference was 32 cm. The placenta weighed 400 g and was noted to be gritty. The baby was found to have a low blood sugar at the time of delivery which responded to a bottled feed. The baby was discharged home 48 h after birth on formula feed. All these comments were contained in the baby's handheld records which the mother had brought with her. The mother cannot remember the last time she attended the local health clinic and cannot recall the name of her health visitor.

There were two other children, one aged 21 years who lived in her own flat and a 3-year-old girl. The father was a lift engineer and had three other children by a previous marriage. The baby's mother thought they were all well.

The problems at presentation were feeding difficulties (the baby was reported to take only 2 ounces every 4–5 h, each feed taking 1 h), coryza and sticky eyes. On examination the child weighed 2.4 kg and her head circumference was 33 cm. She had good tone and appeared alert. The findings of note were a small face with maxillary hypoplasia and a systolic murmur best heard at the left mid and upper sternal edge with fixed splitting of the second heart sound. The rest of her examination was otherwise normal.

She remained in hospital for 3 weeks. In the early part of her admission her poor feeding was confirmed and she was commenced on nasogastric feeding. Additional calories were prescribed after the first week, so that she received a total daily amount of 110 kcal/kg/day, but at the end of her admission she had gained only 110 g.

Haemoglobin	11.5 g/dl
White cell count	$13.7 \times 10^9/l$
Neutrophils	$2.58 \times 10^9/l$
Lymphocytes	$9.93 \times 10^9/l$
Eosinophils	$0.27 \times 10^9/l$
Platelet count	$418 \times 10^9/l$
Serum sodium	135 mmol/l
Serum potassium	4.8 mmol/l
Serum urea	5.4 mmol/l
Serum calcium	2.2 mmol/l
Serum creatinine	54 mmol/l
Serum protein	61 g/dl
Serum albumin	39 g/dl
Serum bicarbonate	24 mmol/l

Serum chloride	103 mmol/l
Serum glucose	5.6 mmol/l
Serum bilirubin	6 µmol/l
Arterial blood gas	Normal
TORCH screen	Normal
Skull X-ray	Normal
Chest X-ray	Normal
Barium studies of upper gastrointestinal tract	Normal
ECG	Normal
Urinary plasma amino acids	Normal
Thyroid function tests	Normal
Sweat test	Normal
Cranial ultrasound	Normal

1. Suggest two further investigations.
2. Suggest a diagnosis.

Paper 9 ANSWERS

Answer 9.1

1. Normal variant

Reject: Duchenne muscular dystrophy
          Benign congenital hypotonia

2. Creatine kinase estimation

Discussion

The child has a normal developmental history when allowance is made for his premature birth. Most paediatricians would feel it appropriate to exclude Duchenne muscular dystrophy in a boy who was not walking at 18 months of age. At 16 months (this child's developmental age), serum creatine phosphokinase estimation could reasonably be delayed but was in reality carried out because of the parents' concern.

Benign hypotonia can be associated with delayed motor milestones but is characterized by a more marked reduction in muscle tone.

Answer 9.2

1. Oesophageal reflux

Discussion

The chest X-ray is normal. The pH probe shows prolonged periods of a drop in oesophageal pH over a 24-h period. This finding suggests gastro-oesophageal reflux; this is a not uncommon cause of apnoeic spells in infancy.

Answer 9.3

1. Immune haemolysis secondary to (i) anti-B in transfused serum or (ii) Gram-negative sepsis
     Non-immune haemolysis from necrotic gut sepsis

Reject: ABO incompatibility

2. Restrict transfusion of group O serum
     Treat sepsis
     Remove necrotic gut if general condition fails to respond to medical management

Discussion

The most likely cause for this infant's hyperbilirubinaemia is immune haemolytic disease resulting from anti-B antibodies in the serum of the transfused group O products. This was exacerbated by the large transfusion requirement.

Gram-negative septicaemia, in particular due to *Clostridia welchii* and *Escherichia coli,* can also result in the production of warm antibody immune haemolysis. In this case with abdominal pathology, infection with these organisms is possible. The positive Coomb's test and blood film findings of agglutination and spherocytes are compatible with either of these causes of non-immune haemolysis.

Answer 9.4

1. Onset of stridor in patients with infantile larynx is almost always within the first 4 weeks of life
   Croup like cough is unusual
   Uncommon for infantile larynx to cause failure of weight gain over a 3 week period
   Stridor is usually inspiratory

2. Haemangioma
   Vascular ring

   Subglottic stenosis
   Vocal cord palsy
   Laryngeal webs
   Cysts, e.g. posterior tongue

   Laryngeal cleft
   Laryngeal papillomas
   Tracheal stenosis

3. Barium oesophagogram/swallow
   Endoscopy

Discussion

In general, infants with persistent stridor should be investigated to establish a precise diagnosis. This may allow appropriate treatment to be planned and an accurate prognosis to be given to the parents. An exception to this may be the normal child with typical features of an infantile larynx in whom symptoms are mild. In these patients, any unusual features should prompt further investigation.

A barium oesophagogram swallow examination should be considered in every infant with persistent stridor, particularly if there is an expiratory component, so that the diagnosis of a vascular ring can be established.

Direct examination of the airways is also indicated in most infants with persistent stidor. Flexible bronchoscopy is ideally suited for the evaluation of such infants because it may be passed through the nose and the entire upper airway examined in addition to the lower airway. The dynamics of the larynx and pharynx may be observed without distortion and the vocal cord movements evaluated. Once the supraglottic structures have been observed the subglottic region and trachea should be examined, even if the cause for the stridor has been located in the supraglottic area.

Other less important examinations in such cases include:

— Radiographs of the neck, especially lateral view with the neck extended, as cystic lesions compressing the respiratory passages may very rarely cause stridor as the only symptom;
— High kilo-voltage filter views of the trachea and bronchi may reveal compression or tracheomalacia;
— MRI of the airway;
— If a vascular ring is suspected following barium swallow and/or endoscopy, cardiac ultrasound and/or angiogram;
— CT scan.

Answer 9.5

1. Chromosomal analysis
Echocardiography
Syphilis serology of mother/baby
HIV identification by polymerase chain reaction or culture of the virus

2. Fetal alcohol syndrome

HIV
Chromosomal disorder

Syphillis

Reject: Feeding difficulties

Discussion

Fetal alcohol syndrome explains the mother's memory loss, the intrauterine growth retardation with hypoglycaemia and poor postnatal growth, along with the features of a small face with hypoplasia of the maxillary region and a cardiac lesion, in this case an atrioseptal defect.

Syphilis may give rise to maxillary hypoplasia and snuffly nose (which on staining the discharge may reveal *Treponema pallidum*). The maternal details of VDRL testing must be sought.

HIV infection is less likely but may be associated with intrauterine growth retardation and poor weight gain, although it does not explain the dysmorphic features. Children presently account for 1% of symptomatic HIV infection; 75% of these case have acquired HIV perinatally from an infected mother. It is said that these children have characteristic facies with a prominent forehead and large eyes. Such children occasionally have lymphadenopathy and hepatomegaly, and may become symptomatic by 1 month of age, presenting with diarrhoea, failure to thrive and opportunistic infection. A definitive diagnosis is made by viral culture or polymerase chain reaction of viral nucleic acid DNA in white blood cells. Finding the p24 viral antigen is highly indicative of infection. IgM levels are not yet reliable and IgG levels reflect placental transfer of antibody although any symptomatic child with antibody should be treated as though infected.

Syndromes with a cardiac anomaly and maxillary hypoplasia include fetal alcohol syndrome, Marfan's syndrome, maternal phenylketonuria, Rubenstein Taybi syndrome, Turner's syndrome and 18 q$^-$.

Paper 10 QUESTIONS

Question 10.1

A 14-year-old West Indian girl was admitted following a first tonic–clonic convulsion. The fit had lasted 20 min and at the time of admission the girl was deeply unconscious but without focal neurological signs. Blood pressure was noted to be raised (200/110 mmHg) immediately after the fit but was normal within 6 h. The remainder of the examination was normal.

Previously the girl had had no significant illnesses. She had two older sisters both of whom were well. She had been brought up by her mother who suffered with hypertension but was otherwise well.

Urea and electrolytes	Normal
Full blood count	Normal (sickle screen negative)
Plasma viscosity	Normal
Liver function tests	Normal
Plasma renin	Normal
Abdominal ultrasound	Normal
VMA screen (urine)	Normal
Cranial CT	Generalized mild cerebral oedema
EEG	Normal

5 days later she was discharged completely well. However, at review on the ward the following week, she complained of severe headaches and was once more hypertensive.

1. What is the diagnosis?
2. Give two investigations you should perform.

Question 10.2

A 41-week-gestation baby was delivered by emergency caesarian section for fetal distress which had been detected by late decelerations in the cardiotocograph and the presence of meconium in the liquor. The baby was delivered covered in meconium. After resuscitation the baby showed increasing tachypnoea with cyanosis and then became apnoeic requiring intubation and ventilation. After initial adjustments to the ventilator settings the following gases were obtained:

pH	7.18
PaO_2	6 kPa

PaCO$_2$ 6 kPa
Base excess   −18 mmol/l

1. What is the likely diagnosis?
2. What is the single most important step during resuscitation of a baby such as this?
3. What three adjustments would you carry out to the ventilator which would improve the baby's condition?
4. What three therapeutic steps should you consider?

Question 10.3

A 7-day-old male Asian infant was admitted with a 24-h history of poor feeding, nasal discharge and mild tachypnoea. He was born at term (birthweight 3 kg) to healthy unrelated parents after an uneventful pregnancy and delivery and had been bottle fed. He had a sister aged 3 years who was well. There was no other history of note.

Examination revealed an unwell infant, with a slight yellow nasal discharge. His respiratory rate was 60 breaths/min, but there were no added sounds in the chest. There were no other specific findings. In view of his poor overall condition, a full septic screen was performed.

Haemoglobin	16.1 g/dl
White cell count	12.5 × 10^9/l
Platelet count	210 × 10^9/l
Sodium	133 mmol/l
Potassium	4.3 mmol/l
Urea	5.1 mmol/l
Glucose	4.1 mmol/l
CSF	0 white cells, 13 red cells, no organisms seen on Gram staining
Urine	3 white cells, no organsims
Chest X-ray	Normal

Pending culture results he was given a broad-spectrum antibiotic. 15 h after admission, his condition deteriorated, with multiple apnoeas. Following ventilation he required large amounts of inotropic support and colloid to maintain adequate blood pressure. He developed a persistent metabolic acidosis, despite several doses of sodium bicarbonate and also became hypoglycaemic. On further examination his peripheral perfusion was reduced, his pulses were difficult to palpate and the liver was palpable 3 cm below the costal margin. All bacterial cultures were negative at this stage.

1. List three possible diagnoses.
2. What three investigations would you perform?

Question 10.4

Following a normal vaginal delivery at term of a healthy 3-kg boy, conjunctivitis was noted at 10 days of age. There was moderate conjunctival infection with a mucopurulent discharge. A swab of the eye was sent to microbiology and the child started on neomycin eye drops. Despite eye drops, conjunctivitis was a problem for the next 3 weeks.

At the age of 7 weeks the child had developed mild tachypnoea and respiratory distress which became worse over a period of 7 days. The child was apyrexial and looked well but had a stacatto cough. Auscultation revealed diffuse crepitations within the chest with slight wheeze. His haemoglobin concentration was normal but the eosinophil count was raised. Immunoglobulins M, G and A were elevated.

Two days later at the beginning of July, a chest X-ray was taken which showed significant hyperexpansion and diffuse bilateral interstitial infiltrates. The child's respiratory difficulty continued for a further 2 months and then started to improve gradually. A very mild conjunctivitis persisted.

There was no history or evidence of gastro-oesophageal reflux and barium swallow, oesophagogram and sweat test were normal.

1. What is the most likely cause of this patient's conjunctivitis?
2. What advice would you give to the parents about the risk to their own health?
3. What is the most likely cause of the child's respiratory problem?

Question 10.5

A 4-year-old Caribbean boy was brought to casualty with a day's history of a painful left hand. On waking he noticed that his hand was starting to swell. At presentation he was unable to flex or extend his fingers, the movements being limited by pain as well as swelling. He had not had any significant trauma to that hand and had otherwise been well.

He was born at full term by normal vaginal delivery in Jamaica and moved to the UK when he was 2 years old. He had not had any illnesses and he had been immunized. He was an only child; his father was a 32-year-old building inspector and his mother a 29-year-old singer.

On examination he was apyrexial. His hand was swollen on the dorsal aspect with generalized tenderness. This area was warm on palpation but there was no apparent cellulitis.

Haemoglobin	8 g/dl
White cell count	6×10^9/l
Platelet count	233×10^9/l

A blood film was performed.

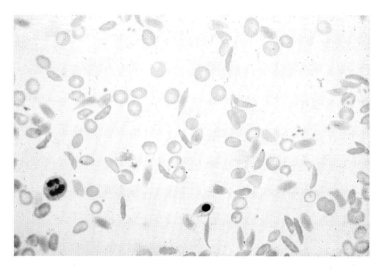

1. Give three abnormalities seen in the blood film.
2. Give a diagnosis.

Paper 10 ANSWERS

Answer 10.1

1. Phaeochromocytoma

Malignant hypertension
Autoimmune disease

2. 24-h urinary catecholamine profile
Specific chromaffin tissue isotope scan (MIBG)

Abdominal CT scan
Blood catecholamine studies (available in some units but not routinely)

Autoantibody screen

Discussion

This girl has evidence of episodic hypertension. The initial findings and investigations do not support a diagnosis of primary renal disease, renal artery stenosis or autoimmune disorder, all of which would be more likely to result in sustained hypertension. Because of the wide variation seen in clinical presentation, autoimmune disease would, however, merit further consideration.

This girl had a phaeochromocytoma which was not detected on any of six 'spot' urinary catecholamine screens because of the episodic nature of the catecholamine release. 24-h catecholamine studies did however reveal a marked excess. Abdominal CT identified a suspicious area in the left adrenal. Diagnosis was confirmed by MIBG scan (an isotope specifically taken up by chromaffin tissue). Histology indicated the tumour to be benign and not typical of the growths seen in the multiple endocrine adenoma syndrome.

Answer 10.2

1. Meconium aspiration syndrome

Persistent fetal circulation
Persistent pulmonary hypertension
Pneumonia

Reject: Respiratory distress syndrome
Transient tachypnoea

2. Aspiration of the pharynx and trachea at the beginning of resuscitation (any answer that does not include this point is incorrect)

3. Increase FiO_2

Increase ventilator rate

Increase peak inspiratory pressure

Prolong expiratory time whilst maintaining rate and mean airway pressure

Reject: Increase I:E ratio

Add PEEP

4. Muscle relaxation

Blood or plasma (if blood pressure sub-optimal)

Antibiotics

Intravenous tolazoline or prostacycline

Intravenous dopamine or dobutamine

Intravenous bicarbonate or THAM

Surfactant

ECMO and nitric oxide

Discussion

The blood gases obtained point to a mixed respiratory and metabolic acidosis. From the history, the most likely explanation for this is meconium aspiration, although pneumonia cannot be excluded. The respiratory distress syndrome is highly unlikely since this is a term baby. Transient tachypnoea rarely produces such profound gas abnormalities. It has been shown that where the possibility of meconium aspiration exists, thorough aspiration of meconium from the pharynx and trachea may diminish the severity of the condition.

Treatment for persistent fetal circulation includes maximal oxygenation so the FiO_2 needs to be sufficient to ensure this occurs. Hyperventilation to drop the $PaCO_2$ to between 3 and 3.5 kPa and hence raising pH may produce secondary pulmonary vasodilation. Increase in peak inspiratory pressure will achieve this and also increase oxygenation. Finally, prolonging the expiratory time may also enhance a drop in $PaCO_2$.

The use of intravenous tolazoline or prostacycline may produce pulmonary vasodilation. Increasing systemic blood pressure by the use of a pressor agent (e.g. dopamine) may also improve pulmonary perfusion by reducing both atrial and ductal shunting. The acidosis needs to be corrected with bicarbonate or THAM and, if necessary, circulating volume maintained with plasma or blood. It is also useful to treat with antibiotics because of the possibility of a secondary bacterial infection. Finally, in order to achieve adequate ventilation, muscle relaxation is usually necessary.

Answer 10.3

1. Viral septicaemia

Left heart outflow tract obstruction (coarctation or critical aortic

stenosis)
Inborn error of metabolism

2. Viral serology, culture and immunofluorescence
Echocardiogram
Serum ammonia and amino acids
Urine organic acid

Discussion

The most likely cause for this form of persentation is infection and a viral aetiology should be considered if bacterial cultures remain negative. This particular infant was found subsequently to have herpes simplex type 1 (HSV-1) on serology and culture. There was no history of herpetic infection in either parent. Any infant presenting with circulatory collapse should also be considered for the possibility of obstructive left-sided heart lesions, in particular coarctation of the aorta and critical aortic stenosis. Both of these lesions will be apparent on echocardiography.

Approximately 70% of babies with neonatal herpes simplex infusion are born to mothers with no history of genital lesions. Neonatal HSV infection may be localized or generalized. It may result in isolated pneumonitis or meningoencephalitis. The prognosis of all but localized infection is poor, and without antiviral treatment about 70% of infants with localized infection will progress to disseminated infection.

Persistent acidosis and hypoglycaemia may be indicative of an inborn error of metabolism. In addition to acute investigations such as serum ammonia and urinary organic acids, liver biopsy and skin fibroblast culture should be taken if possible, should the patient die. The main reason for establishing a diagnosis is to allow later diagnosis using tissue culture and genetic counselling of the family.

Answer 10.4

1. Infection with *Chlamydia trachomatis*

2. To contact their local GP or local genitourinary clinic and be tested for chlamydia as this sexually-transmitted infection may cause non-specific urethritis and infertility if not treated

3. Afebrile pneumonia of infancy (most commonly caused by *Chlamydia trachomatis*)

Ureaplasma urealyticum
Mycoplasma hominus

Bronchiolitis

Discussion

Conjunctivitis secondary to *Chlamydia trachomatis* is very common. It usually occurs 5–14 days after birth and may vary from mild mucoid discharge without significant conjunctival erythema to a profuse discharge, which may be indistinguishable from that associated with *Neisseria gonorrhoea*.

Untreated chlamydial conjunctivitis often resolves spontaneously after several weeks to months. Long-term sequelae are minimal. Ocular carriage of the organism may persist for 2 years.

Gram-stain examination of the ocular discharge is needed and will reveal both polymorphonuclear leucocytes and mononuclear cells. A Giemsa stain and examination of conjunctival scraping containing large numbers of epithelial cells detects chlamydial inclusions in the cytoplasm of the epithelial cells in up to 90% of cases.

Serological evaluation is not useful in the diagnosis of chlamydial conjunctivitis because most infants do not develop IgM antibodies and their antichlamydial IgG is of maternal origin. However, when pneumonia is present, measurement of antichlamydial IgM titre is preferred over nasopharyngeal culture for the diagnosis because it is always elevated when clinical disease is apparent.

Treatment of the mother and her sexual partner with erythromycin or tetracycline for 7–14 days is recommended at the time of diagnosis of the infant's infection. Informing the parents of the possible source of chlamydial infection and the risks to fertility if not treated is mandatory.

Chlamydia trachomatis accounts for up to 70% of afebrile pneumonias occurring in infants from 3–11 weeks of age. The history is typical. Although the total leucocyte count is normal, up to 50% have eosinophil counts >300/mm^3. Serum levels of IgM, IgG and IgA are usually elevated, as in this patient. About 50% of infants will also have middle ear effusions or infection. A diagnosis of bronchiolitis is unlikely in the summer.

Answer 10.5

1. Sickle cells
   Hypochromosia
   Anisocytosis
   Target cells
   Nucleated red blood cells

2. Dactylitis secondary to sickle cell disease
   Sickle cell crisis secondary to osteomyelitis

   Osteomyelitis

Reject: Cellulitis

Discussion

The blood film shows sickled cells as well as variation in size, shape and staining of the red blood cells. Dactylitis is more likely than osteomyelitis as the white cell count is not significantly raised and the child is apyrexial. Antibiotic cover, however, is recommended until the results of blood cultures are available. Cellulitis is excluded as clinically it is not evident.

Paper 11 *QUESTIONS*

Question 11.1

A 4-week-old female infant was referred to clinic by her GP and health visitor because of poor weight gain. The baby was born at 38-weeks gestation after an uneventful pregnancy and a normal vaginal delivery and weighed 3.0 kg. Both parents were 18 years old and had been able to live together only after the birth of the baby when the local authority provided a flat. Until that time, both had lived with their respective parents. Neither the baby's mother nor father were in work.

The health visitor had been closely involved with the family and clearly felt the overall level of care was poor. She had, however, observed the baby to take bottle feeds vigorously on two or three occasions. There was no history of vomiting or diarrhoea. The parents reported that the baby had not grown very well but commented that several members of both families were small.

On examination the child weighed 3.2 kg and looked thin. She was adequately clothed but her clothes were dirty. There was some reddening of the limbs (see picture). There was no nappy rash and she was observed to pass a normal stool. There were no other abnormalities.

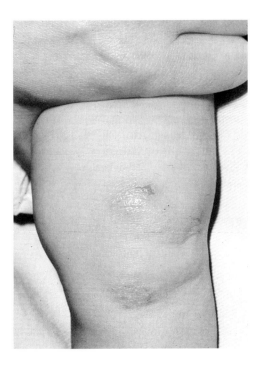

1. What is the diagnosis?
2. What action should be taken?

Question 11.2

A $2\frac{1}{2}$-year-old girl presented at hospital with a 2-week history of lethargy, pallor, pains in her legs and bruising, although there was no overt bleeding. Over the previous 6 months she had had three episodes of tonsilitis and recurrent upper respiratory infections. She was born at 42-weeks gestation and there were no neonatal problems. Her development and general health had been good until this episode began. Her parents were from Nigeria and both were well. There was no family history of sickle cell disease. There were no siblings and she had not taken any drugs in the last 2 months.

On examination she was irritable, pale but afebrile. There were two bruises on her legs but no purpura. There was no sign of infection. Heart rate was 120 beats/min, respiratory rate 30 breaths/min and blood pressure 110/60 mmHg. There was no lymphadenopathy or hepatosplenomegaly. There were no fundal heamorrhages and neurologically she was normal.

Haemoglobin	8.2 g/dl
White cell count	$4.9 \times 10^9/l$
Neutrophils	4%
Lymphocytes	96%
Blood film	No blasts seen, occasional red cell fragments
Platelet count	$156 \times 10^9/l$
Bone marrow aspiration	Hypocellular marrow, no evidence of leukaemic infiltration, no megakaryocytes
Urea and electrolytes	Normal
Liver function tests	Normal
Calcium	Normal
Limb X-rays	Normal
Viral antibody screen	Negative
Haemoglobin electrophoresis	Normal

1. What is the diagnosis?
2. What are three possible causes of this?
3. What two therapeutic measures should you start?

Question 11.3

A 10-month-old caucasian girl was referred for investigation of recurrent chest infections and noisy breathing. She was born at full term, birthweight 3.4 kg after an uneventful pregnancy and delivery. Her parents and 5-year-old brother were well. A heart murmur was noted in the neonatal period, due to severe aortic stenosis with a degree of mitral incompetence. The aortic valve was treated with balloon angioplasty at the age of 6 months, but although this successfully reduced the gradient across the aortic valve, the mitral valve required surgical repair. At the time of referral she was on diuretics and captopril. Her main problems were sweating and tiredness when feeding, noisy breathing both with and between feeds (present since the age of 6 weeks and described as a 'rattling' noise by her parents), vomiting precipitated by coughing, and episodes of frequent offensive stools and abdominal distension.

On examination, her weight was 7.5 kg and her length 71 cm. At rest she had minimal respiratory signs and her cry was normal. Her pulses were of good volume and she had a soft systolic murmur heard best in the aortic area and at the apex. Whilst feeding, however, she became sweaty and developed intercostal recession and stridor, which was much more marked on inspiration than on expiration and was increased by neck flexion. She had a bovine cough.

Chest X-ray	Mild cardiomegaly, lung fields clear
Sweat test	Weight of sweat 118 mg, sodium 14 mmol/l, chloride 8 mmol/l

1. What is the most likely cause of this infant's symptoms?
2. Give three investigations you would perform.

Question 11.4

A 16-year-old boy was referred to hospital because of a serious chest complaint. A week before admission he had consulted his GP complaining of breathlessness which had developed over the previous 2 weeks. During that time he had developed fever and also a cough which was productive of clear sputum only. Although a viral illness was suspected, amoxicillin was prescribed. He had noted increased malaise and had become progressively more short of breath. He was no longer able to go to school or help in the family pet shop. There was no history of chest pain or any other medical history of note. He lived at home and both parents were heavy smokers.

When reviewed by the GP at home, he was sitting up in bed and was alert. However, he was tachypnoeic and centrally cyanosed. He had a sinus tachycardia and a temperature of 37.6°C. Chest auscultation revealed widespread inspiratory crackles throughout both lung fields as the only abnormality. Jugular venous pressure was normal and there was no dependent oedema. There was no finger clubbing, and the teenager was well perfused with a blood pressure of 100/60 mmHg.

When seen in hospital there was little to add to the history. Over the previous week his cough had been essentially non-productive.

Haemoglobin	12 g/dl
White cell count	$13 \times 10^9/l$
ESR	76 mm/h
Arterial blood gases taken in air:	
pH	7.4
PaO_2	5.5 kPa
$PaCO_2$	2.9 kPa
Chest X-ray	Diffuse bilateral, predominantly nodular shadowing
Sputum culture	Negative for growth
Mantoux test 1 in 1000	No induration at 48 h
Blood cultures	Negative
Viral cultures	Negative for influenza A and B, adenovirus, parainfluenzae, myocoplasma pneumoniae, chlamydia psittaci

1. What is the most likely diagnosis?
2. Give two investigations that may help to confirm your diagnosis.

Question 11.5

A 3-week-old child presented with a variety of complaints. She was the fourth offspring of a Turkish Cypriot woman whose second and third pregnancies ended at 30-weeks and 24-weeks gestation by spontaneous abortion in Cyprus. Unfortunately there were no obstetric notes from that time available but the mother knew she was VDRL negative.

The first child was a healthy 5-year-old boy who had phototherapy in the neonatal period. His blood group was B Rhesus positive. The mother was blood group A Rhesus negative and she had a scan at 12 weeks in the fourth pregnancy which showed the fetus to be hydropic. An anomaly scan showed an enlarged liver and spleen. A haemoglobin of 4 g/dl was confirmed by sampling from the umbilical vein and the fetus had fortnightly top-up transfusions, maintaining the haemoglobin between 8 and 14 g/dl.

The baby was born at 34 weeks by emergency caesarian section following an in-utero transfusion which resulted in cord tamponade. The baby was born with Apgar scores of 2 at 1 min and 8 at 5 min. The birthweight was 3.5 kg. Ventilation for 5 days and two doses of surfactant were required. She had two exchange transfusions and two top-up transfusions in the first week and phototherapy was continued for a further week. Her weight fell to 3.2 kg and additional calories were added to her feeds.

In the nursery over the past week she had had persisting diarrhoea. There was candida in the stool. There was no evidence of reducing substances on testing in urine or faeces. She had developed a skin rash which had progressed from a maculopapular eruption to a generalized erythroderma over the past 5 days. Her liver was 3 cm below the right costal margin and her spleen tip was palpable. She had developed a spiking fever; however, all microbiologicial and viral samples (including investigations for HIV and CMV) were negative. Her full blood count, urea and electrolytes, including calcium, phosphate and magnesium, were normal.

1. What is the diagnosis?
2. How has this condition arisen?

Paper 11 *ANSWERS*

Answer 11.1

1. Neglect/insufficient feeding
Psychosocial deprivation

Occult infection, e.g. urinary infection

2. Admit to observe response to feeding, weight gain and social behavior

Call a case conference

Urine microscopy

Discussion

The information presented about this child and the clinical picture are not compatible. The child is failing to thrive despite an apparently good intake without evidence of loss in the form of vomiting or abnormal stool. The social background raises the suspicion of neglect. The observation of single feeds taken well does nothing to confirm the true picture of the child's daily intake. The picture shows reddening of the knees and this may be caused by a reaction to bedding or washing powder; however it can suggest that the child has been left to 'scrabble' in her cot for considerable periods. This case occurred at a time when it was normal practice to nurse infants prone, however red knees and elbows may still be seen in older neglected infants who have learnt to roll, i.e. after 4 months of age.

Under these circumstances the appropriate action is to admit the child for observation. If the child gains weight very rapidly without any other intervention, then this provides strong evidence of neglect. For medicolegal purposes it is essential that all weights are properly documented. This additional evidence (i.e. weight gain in hospital) should be obtained prior to a case conference being called.

It is essential that all possible organic causes for the child's failure to thrive are excluded. No organic cause is indicated from the information provided, however urinary tract infection always merits consideration in these circumstances.

Answer 11.2

1. Hypoplastic anaemia
Congenital aplastic anaemia
Acquired aplastic anaemia

2. Idiopathic
   Virally induced (despite the normal viral titres)
   Hepatitis
   Immune related
   Chemicals/toxins
   Pre-leukaemia

Reject: Drugs
           Schwachman's syndrome

3. Blood transfusion
   Anti-lymphocyte globulin
   Granulocyte transfusion
   Intravenous methylprednisolone
   Antibiotics
   Bone marrow transplant

Discussion

The bone marrow aspiration points to a hypoplastic marrow. Aplastic anaemia has several causes. There is no evidence of previous drug ingestion and she did not have the skeletal features of a Fanconi's anaemia; similarly, there were no features typical of Schwachman's syndrome. Despite the normal viral titres this condition could be virally induced, however, the majority of such cases are idiopathic.

Immediate treatment includes a blood transfusion to correct her anaemia and urgent consideration should be given to an HLA-compatible bone marrow transplant. Other therapeutic options which are less established include anti-lymphocyte globulin and granulocyte transfusions. Febrile illnesses should be treated with broad-spectrum intravenous antibiotics.

Answer 11.3

1. Narrowing of the major airway
   Subglottic stenosis
   Laryngeal web
   Bronchomalacia

Reject: Laryngomalacia

2. Tomograms or penetrated X-rays to show main airways
   Barium swallow
   Bronchoscopy

Discussion

The main problem in this case is chronic stridor. The most common cause for this is laryngomalacia. This however generally presents in the neonatal period and the majority of infants have few associated symptoms and resolve spontaneously. Vocal cord paralysis will also cause stridor, but the cry will be weak if the paralysis is complete. Other causes of stridor in the upper airway include subglottic stenosis, haemangiomas and laryngeal webs. Intrathoracic tracheal narrowing tends to result in expiratory stridor of a wheezing nature and may be associated with feeding problems. Causes include tracheomalacia, tracheal stenosis, tracheo-oesophageal fistula and external compression (e.g. by a vascular ring).

Narrowing of the bronchi may result from bronchomalacia, external compression or foreign bodies. This girl had severe bronchomalacia of the left main bronchus resulting from compression by an enlarged left atrium (secondary to mitral incompetence). Respiratory distress in cardiac disease may result (as in this case) from external compression of the bronchi (usually by the pulmonary artery or left atrium) or from intraluminal changes in the bronchi (e.g. mucosal oedema).

Answer 11.4

1. Bird fancier's lung (extrinsic allergic alveolitis due to an avian protein hypersensitivity)

Influenzae
Viral pneumonia
Tuberculosis
Sarcoidosis
Atypical pneumonia, e.g. mycoplasma or legionaire's disease

Reject: Asthma
Foreign body

2. Estimation of serum precipitating antibody to avian antigens
Intracutaneous injection of extracts of serum and faeces of patient's own bird
Lung biopsy
Gas transfer factor

Angiotensin converting enzyme assay

Discussion

Bird fancier's lung is caused by inhaled avian serum proteins present in the bird's excreta and secreta. It primarily occurs in individuals who breed and keep pigeons. Protein-containing dust is disseminated in the air by birds fluttering their wings during cleaning of pigeon lofts and budgerigar cages.

Acute presentation of extrinsic allergic alveolitis is characteristic of bird fancier's lung. The diagnosis more readily springs to mind when the acute illness follows a clear history of exposure after an interval of 6–8 h. However, there may be no clear-cut temporal relationship.

Many features of this illness may be mimicked by influenza, viral pneumonia, mycobacterium tuberculosis or sarcoidosis. However, none of these diagnoses can account for all the features seen here.

Although both sarcoidosis and mycobacterium tuberculosis may present subacutely with similar chest X-ray results, neither typically produces the amount of breathlessness seen in this child, or the marked impairment of gas exchange.

Answer 11.5

1. Graft-versus-host disease

Congenital immune deficiency syndrome

Reject: CMV infection
HIV infection
Syphilis

2. In-utero transfusion of non-irradiated blood

Discussion

This mother has had severe problems with Rhesus incompatibility. The key clinical features in this child are failure to thrive, progressive skin rash, diarrhoea, hepatomegaly and pyrexia. These are indicative of graft-versus-host disease.

Graft-versus-host disease is largely seen in immunosuppressed children, e.g. those who have had bone marrow transplantation. However, in this child it may have arisen either as a consequence of intrauterine transfusion with non-irradiated blood (as the fetus has a relatively poorly developed immune system) or may be associated with an inherited immunodeficiency state. There are no additional features to support the diagnosis of an inherited defect.

Paper 12 QUESTIONS

Question 12.1

A 2-year-old girl was brought to casualty having been found at home unconscious. She was discovered in a bedroom by her mother who thought initially that the child was asleep. The child had been completely well prior to the incident. In the past she had been seen in casualty on three occasions following accidents at home. There was no significant perinatal history.

There were three older children in the family which was well known to social services. The mother had had a series of partners in the past 10 years, was of limited mental ability and was epileptic. General concern about the children had in the past led to two case conferences being held. Both had concluded the family was 'chaotic but caring'.

On examination the child was pink, well perfused, breathing normally and apyrexial. She was unkempt but well nourished. There were bruises on her legs but no other injuries. She responded only to painful stimuli. Her fundi were normal and there were no focal neurological signs. The remainder of the examination was normal.

1. Give two diagnoses.
2. Give the most important investigation to perform.

Question 12.2

A 12-h-old neonate suddenly developed cyanosis, breathlessness and vomiting. On examination there was peripheral cyanosis, a heart rate of 280 beats/min (see ECG overleaf) and a palpable liver, 4 cm below the right costal margin. A chest X-ray was obtained, which was normal.

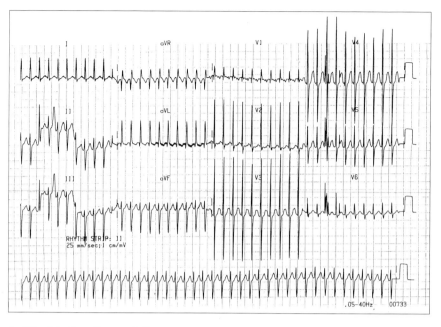

1. What is the diagnosis?
2. What is your immediate treatment – give two possible approaches?

Question 12.3

A 3-year-old girl presented with a 6-month history of episodic loss of consciousness followed by generalized tonic–clonic convulsions. These occurred at any time of the day and had no obvious precipitating cause. There was no past medical history of note and despite these episodes her development was within normal limits and she was not regressing. Her parents had recently separated and her mother was being treated with antidepressants. In the family history, a cousin living abroad was said to have a similar problem and a paternal uncle died suddenly in his teens from unknown causes.

Examination revealed a well-grown child with no detectable abnormalities. Developmental assessment was also entirely normal. Several EEG recordings were performed, including following sleep deprivation over a 24-h period, all of which were normal. Other investigations including serum electrolytes, calcium, magnesium, full 'metabolic screen' and brain CT scan were all normal. A trial of anticonvulsant therapy reduced the tonic–clonic movements, but the episodes of loss of consciousness persisted unchanged.

1. Suggest a possible cause for these episodes.
2. What investigation would you perform?

Question 12.4

A 7-year-old child presented to hospital with his third severe asthmatic attack. He was treated with regular nebulized ß-2 agonists and intravenous aminophylline. Due to his respiratory difficulty and pain on swallowing due to apthos ulcers in his mouth, he was given an intravenous infusion (dextrose 4%/saline 0.18%). Thirty-six h later wheeze and recession were still moderately severe. His oxygen saturation in air was 91% and he was apyrexial. At this stage blood was taken.

Haemoglobin	13 g/dl
White cell count	$9 \times 10^9/l$
Sodium	123 mmol/l
Potassium	4.5 mmol/l
Urine microscopy	No abnormal findings
Urine osmolality	600 mmol/kg
Chest X-ray 36 h after admission	Considerable hyperinflation but no other abnormality

1. What two changes to his management would you propose?
2. What is the most likely cause of his hyponatraemia?

Question 12.5

A 7-year-old boy whose parents were first cousins attended the outpatient department with a 6-month history of recurrent abdominal pain and arthralgia. The episodes had worsened and were now occurring daily. His appetite had decreased but his bowel habits and appearance had not altered. His school performance had declined. He said he was being bullied at school. He also complained that he could not clearly see written text when displayed using an overhead projector.

His parents also expressed concern regarding his vision. He denied the use/abuse of any drugs or medicines but remarked that his mother and father were considering getting divorced.

On examination he appeared well but was dribbling saliva from the left corner of his mouth. He had a very expressionless face and had early signs of cataract development in his left eye. Otherwise examination was unremarkable with no evidence of papilloedema or peripheral neuropathy. Blood pressure in his right arm was 110/65 mmHg. All his joints had a normal range of movements and function. Urine analysis showed a large quantity of protein and no glucose. A cranial CT and EEG were normal.

1. Give a diagnosis.
2. What two investigations would you think appropriate?

Paper 12 *ANSWERS*

Answer 12.1

1. Ingestion of anticonvulsants

Non-accidental injury

Encephalitis

'Metabolic disorder', e.g. Reye's syndrome

2. Toxicology screen
Rapid 'stick' blood glucose estimation

Skeletal survey
Cranial CT scan

Urea and electrolytes
Liver function tests
Full blood count
Urine and plasma amino acids
Ammonia
Blood glucose
Lumbar puncture
Blood culture
Urine culture

Discussion

The history points to an ingestion of the mother's anticonvulsant tablets. In this 'chaotic' family the anticonvulsants may well have been accessible and in addition the child is unlikely to have been closely supervised. However, physical abuse cannot be excluded on the evidence given and must be considered. It is important not to be swayed by the previous case conference conclusions.

There is little to suggest any form of disease process; however, in reaching this conclusion the history must be interpreted with caution. It is likely in a family such as the one described that early signs of significant illness might well be missed. As a result there may well have been a prodromal phase of, for example, Reye's syndrome without anyone having noticed.

Answer 12.2

1. Supraventricular tachycardia

Reject: Ventricular tachycardia
              Sinus tachycardia
              Nodal tachycardia

2. DC shock
   Facial immersion in cold water
   Intravenous adenosine
   Intravenous fleccainide
   Intravenous verapamil

Discussion

Supraventricular tachycardia is an important cause of cardiogenic shock and heart failure in infancy. It is potentially fatal and should be treated urgently. The distinction between supraventricular tachycardia and sinus tachycardia is determined by the rate. The upper limit of heart rate in a neonate with an appropriate sinus tachycardia is 220 beats/min, whereas supraventricular tachycardia usually develops at heart rate >270 beat/min. This frequently needs to be confirmed by a formal ECG.

There are various medical treatments for supraventricular tachycardia. While verapamil has been suggested as first-line treatment there is the potential for asystole and consequently the safest treatment is facial immersion in cold water. Recently, intravenous adenosine or fleccinide have been suggested as a safe alternative.

Answer 12.3

1. Cardiac dysrhythmia
   Idiopathic long QT syndrome

   Epilepsy

2. ECG (following exercise)

Discussion

Prolongation of the Q–T interval occurs in Jervell and Lange-Nielsen syndrome (showing autosomal recessive inheritance with associated deafness) and Romano–Ward syndrome (autosomal dominant without deafness). Typically, presentation is with recurrent syncope, associated seizure activity resulting from haemodynamic collapse. Sudden death from ventricular fibrillation is common and in untreated patients with symptoms a mortality rate of >70% in 15 years has been reported. Patients with this condition differ from normal in that their Q–T interval does not shorten after exercise, and indeed a resting ECG may not reveal the diagnosis. Recently, genetic markers for this condition have been identified on the short arm of chromosome 11 (11p).

A young patient, as in this case, would be unable to describe symptoms suggesting a cardiac cause for these episodes (dizzyness, lightheadedness, blackouts). However, the history of syncope preceding convulsions and the response of the seizure activity to anticonvulsants with no effect on the syncopal attacks themselves, coupled with the family history of sudden death are suggestive of a cardiac cause.

Epilepsy as a primary diagnosis is less likely given the normal EEG and clear family history, but is not completely excluded.

Answer 12.4

1. Addition of steroid therapy
Restriction of intravenous fluids

Addition of ipratropium bromide

Reject: Bronchoscopy

2. Excessive antidiuretic hormone release

Discussion

Treatment of a severe asthmatic attack involves administration of ß-2 agonists, usually in the form of nebulized salbutamol and steroid, usually as oral prednisolone or intravenous hydrocortisone. Oxygen saturation should be measured and oxygen given as required. Nebulizers should be run on oxygen. If the child shows no improvement or deteriorates, nebulized salbutamol may be increased in frequency and intravenous administration commenced of either aminophylline or salbutamol. There is a theoretical advantage of using an anticholinergic agent (i.e. ipratropium bromide) — which acts on muscarinic receptors distributed mainly in central airways, in addition to a ß-2 agonist (i.e. salbutamol) — which acts on ß-2 receptors in the peripheral airways. However, there is little clinical evidence of enhanced bronchodilatation when these drugs are used in combination.

Many disease states, medications and pathophysiological processes can alter antidiuretic hormone secretion. In some of these, antidiuretic hormone release may be mediated by stimulation of volume receptors, as in the decreased venous return produced by positive pressure ventilation in severe asthma.

Answer 12.5

1. Wilson's disease

Reject: Behavioural disorder
            Subacute sclerosing panencephalitis
            Cerebral tumour
            Epilepsy
            Neurodegenerative disorders
            Hypothyroidism
            Systemic lupus erythematosis

2. Serum caeruloplasmin
    Urinary copper
    Serum copper
    Penicillamine challenge

Discussion

The salient features are the deterioration in school performance, the drooling, alteration in vision with cataract formation and proteinuria. Attributing the cause of his academic decline to a behavioural disorder does not fit in with the overall clinical picture. A history of domestic altercations does not explain his clinical condition. The abuse of solvents and other noxious agents are denied. Other causes include neurological problems such as subacute sclerosing panencephalitis, cerebral tumour, epilepsy and degenerative disorders. These are unlikely as the CT and EEG are normal. Epilepsy would be unlikely to give rise to a fixed expressionless appearance. Hypothyroidism is associated with failing at school but does not give rise to the other clinical features here. Systemic lupus erythematosis is not associated with cataracts and the systemic blood pressure is normal.

Wilson's disease can have a range of central nervous system manifestations from peripheral neuropathy to frank psychiatric conditions such as acute psychosis. Basal ganglia changes may not show on cranial CT.

Proteinuria is seen in tubular disorders such as: primary renal tubular acidosis, cystinosis, Lowe's syndrome, galactosaemia, Ehlers–Danlos syndrome, diabetes mellitus, adrenal dysfunction and Wilson's disease. Of these conditions, cataract formation is seen in Lowe's syndrome, galactosaemia, diabetes mellitus and Wilson's disease.

Lowe's syndrome is usually diagnosed in infancy with marked hypotonia and congenital cataracts with progressive severe mental retardation. Galactosaemia similarly presents in infancy. Diabetes can cause abdominal pain and cataract formation but more commonly has an acute onset in childhood. The urine is clear on testing for glucose.

Paper 13 *QUESTIONS*

Question 13.1

A pregnant woman presented at 34-weeks gestation following a spontaneous rupture of the membranes. It was decided that labour should be allowed to proceed. The infant was delivered vaginally, without assistance, 43 h later. The baby was born in good condition with Apgar scores of 9 at 1 min and 10 at 5 min. Birthweight was 2.6 kg. The baby was admitted to the special care nursery because of prematurity. 14 h later and immediately following a feed, the child was noted to be blue with raised respiratory rate.

This was the first child in the family and he was conceived after several attempts at in-vitro fertilization. Both parents were healthy. The child's father was an RAF pilot.

On examination the child was peripherally and centrally cyanosed. The respiratory rate was raised at about 100 breaths/min. There were no added sounds on listening to the lungs. Femoral pulses were easily felt and the liver was palpable 3 cm below the costal margin. There was an obvious systolic murmur loudest at the left sternal edge.

Arterial blood gas in air:
pH   7.21
PaO_2 3.1 kPa
$PaCO_2$ 4.1 kPa

The chest X-ray showed clear lung fields and heart of normal size.

1. What is the diagnosis?
2. Give three investigations you should perform?

Question 13.2

A 14-year-old boy was referred to clinic. He had been 'chesty' since the age of 7 years and had been treated for pneumonia on three occasions since then. Over the past 4 months his cough had become more productive and he was producing up to a teaspoonful of green sputum daily. Over the past year he had become more breathless on exertion and despite a normal appetite had lost several kilograms in weight. His stools were occasionally loose. He had smoked 1–2 cigarettes/day between the age of 12 and 13 years, but had not smoked since then.

On examination he was pale and thin and had finger clubbing. His chest was clear on auscultation and did not appear to be hyperinflated. Abdominal examination was normal. A moist cough was heard during examination. Chest X-ray showed hyperinflation and widespread bronchial wall thickening. Lung function tests showed a moderate obstructive ventilatory defect. A full immunological review, including immunoglobulins and subclasses, showed no abnormality. The following results were available from his GP:

Haemoglobin	9.1 g/dl
MCV	66 fl
MCH	23 pg
MCHC	28 g/dl
Blood film	Hypochromic and microcytic changes
Serum ferritin	380 µg/l (normal up to 150 µg/l)
Free erythrocyte protoporphyrin	12 µg/g haemoglobin (normal <3 µg/g)
Serum iron	6 µmol/l
Total iron binding capacity	24 µmol/l
Transferrin saturation	25%

1. What is the most likely underlying diagnosis?
2. Give two investigations that may confirm the underlying diagnosis.
3. What is your interpretation of his blood results?

Question 13.3

A 10-day-old female Asian infant was admitted with a 1-day history of lethargy and poor feeding. She was born at term (birthweight 3.2 kg) to healthy parents who were first cousins. They had another girl aged 3 years who was well. Prior to the last 24 h she had been feeding well and had had an adequate urine output.

On examination she was apyrexial and moderately dehydrated. Her weight was 2.85 kg. She was floppy and disliked being handled. There was no abnormal skin pigmentation and her external genitalia were normal. Her blood pressure was 130/95 mmHg in both arms and 130/90 mmHg in both legs. Sepsis was suspected and a full infection screen was performed before she was treated with antibiotics.

Heamoglobin	14.7 g/dl
White cell count	9.5×10^9/l
Platelet count	247×10^9/l
Serum sodium	120 mmol/l
Serum potassium	13.8 mmol/l
Serum urea	15.9 mmol/l
Urine sodium	131 mmol/l

Urine potassium	11.7 mmol/l
Urine urea	211 mmol/l
Urine osmolality	520 mOsmol/l
Urine pH	5
Arterial gas pH	7.22
Arterial gas $PaCO_2$	3.6 kPa
Arterial gas PaO_2	12.1 kPa
Renal ultrasound	Kidneys and urinary tract normal
CSF	Normal microscopy and biochemistry
Urine microscopy	Normal

1. What is the likely diagnosis?
2. What two investigations would you perform to confirm this?

Question 13.4

A 5-year-old girl was admitted after presenting with two episodes of generalized convulsions. Each convulsion consisted of pain in both arms and legs following which her arm twitched for about 30 s and then her legs for a similar period. The second episode occurred 10 min after the first. She was apyrexial at this time and did not lose consciousness. She was continent of anal and uretral sphincters. There was no previous history of fitting or convulsions and no family history of note.

The parents had noticed that her behaviour had changed over the past 10 months, since the birth of her sister. Her mother described her as a monster now compared to an angel prior to her sister's birth. Her school was worried about her performance in general. She was noted to have a poor attention span. She had also been picking at the paint on the pipes in her bedroom and she wanted her room redecorated. The family lived in a three-bedroom maisonette converted from an Edwardian house. She started to walk at 14 months, after sitting at 6 months and started school at 5 years.

On examination she appeared well and happy. Neurologically she had normal fine and gross motor movements, which she demonstrated without difficulty. She had a normal gait and no evidence of cerebellar signs. Her cranial nerves were intact and her pupils were equal and reactive to light. Her fundi could not be seen as she became weary of being examined and no longer cooperated.

1. Suggest four appropriate diagnoses and give appropriate fundoscopic changes for each condition.

Question 13.5

An infant was delivered by caesarian section at 35-weeks gestation. Liquor was normal. The infant was transferred to the postnatal ward and was noted to be tachypnoeic at the age of 4 h. The child was apyrexial and pink in air with mild intercostal recession but normal air entry over both left and right lung fields. Heart sounds were normal, nasal passages patent and there were no obvious dysmorphic features. A nasogastric tube passed easily into the stomach.

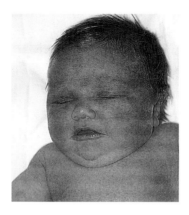

1. How can you explain the child's appearance?
2. What is the likely diagnosis of the respiratory problem?

The child became increasingly unwell and a cranial ultrasound was performed which was normal. The following ECG rhythm strip was obtained.

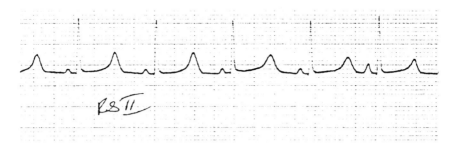

3. What is the most likely cause of the changes seen in this rhythm strip?

The baby required ventilation and was monitored by a continuous ECG trace. Occasionally the ECG trace became abnormal but then reverted back to its previous pattern. One of the abnormal sections of the ECG trace was captured and is shown opposite.

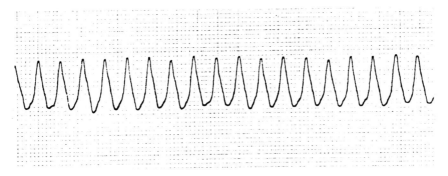

4. What is your interpretation of this ECG rhythm?

5. What three other problems do you think this child may develop?

Paper 13 *ANSWERS*

Answer 13.1

1. Cyanotic congenital heart disease
Persistent fetal circulation
Sepsis

Reject: Aspiration
 Respiratory distress syndrome

2. Echocardiogram
ECG
Infection screen
Blood culture
Lumbar puncture
Nitrogen washout test

Full blood count
Urine culture
Cardiac catheter

Serum urea and electrolytes
C-reactive protein

Discussion

This child has cyanotic congenital heart disease; in this particular case, transposition of the great vessels. The presentation is also compatible with persistent fetal circulation, which may result from various insults. However, in this child, respiration seems to have been well established at birth and therefore some later event, such as sepsis or aspiration, needs to be considered as a possible antecedent to the establishment of presistent fetal circulation. The prolonged rupture of membranes further supports the possibility of infection. Although the initial deterioration followed a feed, the clear X-ray virtually excludes an aspiration episode of sufficient severity to cause the child's current problems.

The description is quite unlike respiratory distress syndrome.

Answer 13.2

1. Cystic fibrosis

  Bronchiectasis follwing severe pneumonia
  Primary ciliary dyskinesia
  Bronchiectasis follwing foreign body aspiration
  Bronchomalacia
  Lobarsequestration

2. Sweet test
  Genotypic analysis looking for common mutations found in patients with cystic fibrosis

  Sputum culture
  Ciliary function and ultrastructure
  Bronchoscopy
  Chest CT scan
  Mantuox test

3. Anaemia associated with chronic infection

Discussion

The long history of chest problems, finger clubbing, loose stools, bronchial wall thickening on chest X-ray, an obstructive ventilatory defect and normal immunity make cystic fibrosis by far the most likely diagnosis. Primary ciliary dyskinesia is less common (1 in 16 000) and usually presents with respiratory symptoms from the neonatal period. Sinusitis and ear infections are also common. Pneumonia, foreign body and sequestration are unlikely due to the widespread changes on X-ray. Bronchomalacia usually presents at an earlier age.

The genotype of patients with cystic fibrosis can now be determined in about 80% of cases in the UK. However, the sweat test remains the definitive test for the diagnosis of cystic fibrosis. Any patient with a recurrent productive cough should be considered for a sweat test as part of their diagnostic work up.

Other causes of suppurative lung disease are:

Widerspread:	Focal:
Idiopathic	Lung collapse
Primary ciliary dyskinesia	Bronchial obstruction: foreign body,
Immune deficiency	stenosis, tumour
Inhalation	Parenchymal abnormality: lung cyst,
Bronchomalacia	lobar sequestration

The blood results suggest an anaemia associated with chronic infection. Treatment with iron may be ineffective. The mild anaemia associated with chronic infections and inflammation may be normochromic or hypochromic and microcytic. In this situation, standard tests of iron deficiency may be difficult to interpret. Serum ferritin is probably the most useful. It is low in iron deficiency and usually increased in anaemia or chronic disease. The iron and total iron-binding capacity are of little value because of suppression of the transferrin level and the rapid fall in the serum iron as a result of the inflammation. Likewise, the free erythrocyte protoporphyrin is usually raised.

Answer 13.3

1. Pseudohypoaldosteronism
   18-oxidation defect

   Congenital adrenal hyperplasia

Reject: Renal tubular acidosis

2. Plasma renin activity
   Aldosterone level

Discussion

The diagnosis of pseudohypoaldosteronism is suggested by urinary salt washing, hypertension, non-virilized genitalia and gross hyperkalaemia in the presence of apparently normal renal structure concentrating ability. The plasma electrolytes are similar to those found in 18-oxidation defects, but in pseudohypoaldosteronism the plasma renin activity and aldosterone levels are massively elevated and aldosterone metabolites in the urine are raised.

The condition arises from renal tubular unresponsiveness to aldosterone, possibly as a result of a reduced Na^+/K^+-ATPase in the renal tubule. Inheritance is autosomal recessive, although a dominant type has been reported. Males with this condition may masquerade as congenital adrenal hyperplasia. Treatment is with sodium chloride supplementation (the requirements may be extremely large in the first years of life), which expands the extracellular fluid volume. Tubular flow and delivery of solute to the distal nephron is increased, resulting in a favourable gradient for potassium secretion. This occurs despite little or no mineralocorticoid stimulation of potassium secretion. The amount of supplementation required may decrease as a result of proximal tubular maturation and the tendency of the child to ingest more salt.

Answer 13.4

1. Papilloedema intoxication/   Lead
    hydrocephalus

    Optic atrophy   Metachromatic leukodystrophy
                                Batten's disease

    Cherry-red spot   Niemann-Pick type C disease

    Pale macula with retinal   Juvenile amaurotic idiocy form of
       pigmentation   lipofuscinosis (Spielmeyer-Sjögren
                                syndrome)

Discussion

The question asks for lesions associated with a progressive dementing disorder. Lead intoxication may be a suggestion given the age of the house and the picking of the paint. Hydrocephalus may also present with dementia and papilloedema. Metachromatic leukodystrophy may just present with psychiatric manifestations, although more commonly the initial stages show a loss of reflexes secondary to accompanying peripheral neuropathy. Myoclonic episodes, dementia and optic atrophy are seen in Batten's disease, which is one of the commoner dementing conditions. Ganglion cells are enlarged with lipofuscin material. Niemann–Pick type C disease can present as a neuropsychiatric disorder. There is increased sphingomyelin and cholesterol in visceral organs and characteristic foam cells in the bone marrow. Spielmeyer–Sjögren syndrome tends to present with reduced visual acuity followed by fits and psychomotor regression. Spasticity, dystonia and eventual akinesia develop.

Answer 13.5

1. Infant of a diabetic mother

2. Idiopathic respiratory distress syndrome
    Pneumonia due to Group B haemolytic streptococcus
    Transient tachypnoea of the newborn

Reject: Meconium aspiration syndrome

3. Hypocalcaemia

    Myocarditis, rheumatic or viral
    Long Q–T syndrome, Jervell and Lange–Nielsen or
       Romano–Ward syndrome
    'Drugs' e.g. procainamide

4. Ventricular tachycardia

Reject: Sinus tachycardia
          Atrial tachycardia
          Supraventricular tachycardia

5. Increased risk of congenital malformation
   Transient tachypnoea of the newborn
   Increased hypocalcaemia and jaundice
   Polycythaemia
   Hypertrophic cardiomyopathy
   Renal vein thrombosis
   Birth complications can ensue including asphyxia and shoulder dystocia

Discussion

The first ECG trace was taken from a child whose blood sugar was low. The heart rate of 120 beats/min is normal for a neonatal patient. The Q–T interval, however, is abnormally long for the heart rate. The ST segment appears particularly prolonged which suggests hypocalcaemia. This is a complication of an infant of a diabetic mother. Hypocalcaemia only affects the duration of the ST segment.

Ventricular tachycardia is a series of premature ventricular contractions at a rate of between 120 and 180/min. Ventricular tachycardia is rare in children but is a serious arrhythmia and may signify myocardial damage or dysfunction. It can deteriorate to ventricular fibrillation, although this is not as likely as in an adult with coronary artery disease. Complete abolition of the arrhythmia is less important than keeping the rate below 150/min for infants.

Paper 14 *QUESTIONS*

Question 14.1

A 10-year-old Asian girl presented to outpatients with a 1-month history of recurrent headaches. Each headache usually lasted no more than 2 h and was eased by paracetamol. The headache was mainly left-sided but occasionally affected the right side. The headaches were often accompanied by nausea and on a few occasions the child had vomited. The attacks were most often present on waking in the morning and were noted both on weekdays and weekends.

Both parents were well but did suffer from infrequent headaches. The maternal grandmother was known to have severe migraine. There was a younger brother, aged 5 years, who suffered from asthma. There was no significant past medical history.

On examination she was well grown and was intellectually normal. Throughout the systems, nothing abnormal was detected; in particular, both fundi were normal and blood pressure was 110/65 mmHg. On the CT scan, there was no intracranial pathology.

1. What is the diagnosis?
2. What is the most appropriate treatment?

Question 14.2

A 10-year-old Afro-Caribbean boy was admitted to hospital having been found by his grandparents confused, lethargic and unable to answer questions. The previous day he complained of headache after returning from fishing, and had gone to bed early. There was no history of head injury, fits, change in school performance or ingestion of drugs and he had never had a similar episode.

He was normally looked after by his grandparents, his parents having died when he was $2\frac{1}{2}$ years of unknown cause. He was born at 28-weeks gestation and had been ventilated. His subsequent development was normal and apart from an orchidopexy he had never had any medical problems. He had been to Jamaica on holiday 6 months previously. His grandparents were being treated with amiodarone and non-steroidal anti-inflammatory medications.

On examination his pulse was 66 beats/min, blood pressure 135/85 mmHg and he was afebrile. His oxygen saturation in air was 99%. He was confused, but making random spontaneous movements, opening his eyes and withdrawing in response to pain. His Glasgow coma scale was 10. His pupils were 4 mm in diameter, reacting normally directly and consensually. The fundi were normal, there was no facial asymmetry and he had a normal gag reflex. Power and tone were normal in all limbs; the reflexes were generally decreased but present in all limbs and the plantar responses were equivocal.

There was no neck stiffness.

Haemoglobin	14.5 g/dl
White blood cells	13.4×10^9/l
Neutrophils	20%
Lymphocytes	70%
Platelet count	309×10^9/l
Haemoglobin electrophoresis	HbAA
Glucose	7.8 mmol/l

1. What are the three most likely diagnoses?
2. Give the three investigations which you consider most important to perform now.
3. How would you treat him immediately?

Question 14.3

An 8-year-old Indian boy was admitted with a 2-week history of diarrhoea, pyrexia and muscular weakness. He was born in the UK and had no significant past medical history. All his immunizations were complete. He had spent the last 7 months visiting relatives in a small village in India, and returned to England 5 days previously. The illness began with pyrexia and frequent loose stools. After several days he complained of pain behind the knees and in his elbows. He then developed weakness in his legs, followed by his arms. He had a poor urinary stream, noted by his parents.

On examination he looked thin and had multiple skin lesions compatible with mosquito bites. He was apyrexial. Cardiovascular, respiratory and abdominal examination were unremarkable. His visual fields were normal to confrontation, and his cranial nerves were symmetrical and normal, with no evidence of bulbar involvement. He had marked weakness of neck flexion and in the small muscles of the hands. He could not tense his abdominal muscles. He had a lumbar lordotic posture and a waddling gait. In his lower limbs he had a generalized reduction in power, more marked distally, and foot drop. Reflexes were normal in the arms and reduced in the legs. All sensory modalities appeared intact, but his coordination was slightly impaired.

Haemoglobin	11.5 g/dl
White cell count	10.8×10^9/l
Platelet count	517×10^9/l
Blood film	Normal red cells, no malarial parasites
Serum electrolytes	Normal
Liver function	Normal
Creatine kinase	102 IU/l (normal 25–200 IU/l)

Heavy metal screen	Normal
Porphyrin screen	Normal
CSF microscopy	0 red cells, 0 white cells, protein 0.2 g/l, no organisms
CSF culture	No growth
Stool culture	Campylobacter sp., giardia cysts
Stool virology	Negative

1. What is the most likely diagnosis?
2. What is the next investigation you would perform?

Question 14.4

A 14-year-old boy was referred because of breast enlargement. This had been increasing gradually and he was now being teased and bullied at school. He was very thin and this made his gynaecomastia more obvious. He had not received any form of drug over the preceding months.

On examination he had 6 cm diameter of breast tissue on either side which appeared slightly tender. There was no galactorrhoea. Pubertal development was Tanner stage 3 and his testes measured 14 ml in volume on both sides.

Haemoglobin	13×10^9/l
White cell count	12×10^9/l
Urea and electrolytes	Normal
Karyotype	46 XY
Serum luteinizing hormone	1.2 U/l (normal 0.8-8.7 U/L)
Follicle stimulating hormone	4.9 U/l (normal 0.6-4.9 U/L)
Plasma testosterone	22 nmol/l (normal 10-30 nmol/l)
Oestradiol	170 pmol/l (normal <250 pmol/l)
Serum prolactin	80 mU/l (normal <420 mU/l)
Bone age	14 years
Liver function tests	Normal

1. What is the most likely diagnosis of this 14-year-old boy's gynaecomastia?
2. What is the natural history of this boy's gynaecomastia?
3. Give three other causes of gynaecomastia occurring at this age.

Question 14.5

An 11-month-old boy presented with a history of passing red-coloured urine on alternate days for the past 2 weeks. There was no history of trauma and he had remained well throughout this episode. In the family history an uncle died of renal tuberculosis 20 years ago. The boy was not receiving any medication. He was an only child of West Indian parents; his father was a 34-year-old tax inspector and his mother a 31-year-old shoe designer. The boy had not travelled out of the UK.

On examination the boy was not pale and was apyrexial. His abdomen was soft with no hepatosplenomegaly and no palpable masses. His urethral meatus appeared normal and his blood pressure in the right arm was 85/45 mmHg. There was no proteinuria on testing.

Haemoglobin	11.6 g/dl
White cell count	16.8×10^9/l
Platelet count	499×10^9/l
Serum sodium	136 mmol/l
Serum potassium	4.5 mmol/l
Serum urea	8.0 mmol/l
Serum creatinine	53 mmol/l
Serum protein	53 mmol/l
Serum albumin	31 mmol/l
Serum bicarbonate	25 mmol/l
Serum chloride	103 mmol/l

1. What three further points of family history are required?
2. What three further investigations are required?

Paper 14 ANSWERS

Answer 14.1

1. Migraine

Tension headache

Visual abnormality

Reject: Brain tumour

2. Simple analgesics
Simple analgesics plus separate antiemetic, e.g. prochlorperazine
Pizotifen

Clonidine

Reject: Propranolol
Ergot-containing compounds

Discussion

This child has significant headaches and the history and examination raise the possibility of a brain tumour with secondary hydrocephalus. The CT scan revealed neither lesion and therefore other causes must be considered. The child in fact proved to have migraine and the history largely supports this diagnosis. Whilst the recurrent headaches seen in true migraine are never exclusively confined to a single side, a predominance may well be seen. The early morning nature of the headaches here is unusual. From the information available, these pains could result from tension headaches and similarly ocular problems have not been positively excluded. Nasal symptoms are not mentioned, however any existing sinus problems are likely to have been revealed by the CT scan.

Current treatment in this girl is already largely successful in that the attacks are contained to a duration of 2 h. Vomiting is still a problem and the addition of a simple antiemetic is likely to be of benefit.

Answer 14.2

1. Viral encephalitis
   Bacterial meningitis
   Drug ingestion
   Intracerebral bleed

   Head trauma
   Reye's syndrome

   Organic acidaemia
   Space-occupying lesion
   Hepatic failure

2. Cerebral CAT scan
   EEG
   Drug screen
   Urea and electrolytes
   Blood culture
   Plasma ammonia
   Liver function tests
   Urinary organic and amino acids

3. Intravenous broad-spectrum antibiotics
   Intravenous acyclovir
   Intravenous mannitol
   Intravenous glucose infusion
   Fluid restriction
   Dexamethasone
   Anticonvulsants

Discussion

This boy has a significant encephalopathy and this history represents a not uncommon clinical problem. In this age group, encephalitis is the most likely explanation, although meningtis is possible (and in clinical practice, particularly so if the patient has already received antibiotics). The change in conscious level and the absence of fever and neck stiffness make a meningitis rather less likely.

The raised white cell count favours an infectious cause for his change in level of consciousness rather than a chemical cause. Drug ingestion and a metabolic cause are both important in the differential diagnosis. Infection may precipitate decompensation in patients with an underlying metabolic disorder. The first presentation of an inborn error would be unusual at this age but some less severe disorders, particularly urea cycle abnormalities, may become apparent this late in life. The relatively sudden onset is consistent with an intracerebral bleed (e.g. from an aneurysm) but some degree of laterality would be more usual. There has been no clear history of trauma and as he was rational the previous day and there are no signs of trauma this is unlikely. He does not have sickle cell anaemia or diabetes. He is older than usual for Reye's syndrome and this history (without significant preceding illness or vomiting) is not typical. Finally, a space-occupying lesion, e.g. a cerebral abscess or tumour, may be present in this way and must therefore be excluded.

The most important feature in considering investigation is to avoid a lumbar puncture in the presence of altered consciousness; although the fundi are normal, papilloedema may not be seen even in the presence of raised intracranial pressure. If it is felt essential to obtain a sample of CSF, a cranial CAT scan should be arranged first. A CAT scan will demonstrate the presence of space-occupying lesions, cerebral oedema, possible localization of an encephalitis to the temporal lobe suggesting a Herpes simplex encephalitis, an intracerebral bleed and possibly evidence of trauma.

Blood gases are important in any critically ill child and here may help in diagnosing a metabolic disorder as well as indicating the need for correction of an acidosis. A drug screen (normally urine) is essential to identify drug ingestion and a serum ammonia estimation will identify either Reye's syndrome, liver failure or an inborn error causing hyperammonaemia. Finally, an EEG will identify encephalitis.

It is essential to cover the possibility of meningitis at the earliest opportunity with a broad-spectrum antibiotic. Similarly, pending the results of a scan or EEG, there is evidence that early treatment with acyclovir will improve the outcome of herpes encephalitis. Intravenous mannitol will help reduce cerebral oedema and may produce improvement in the conscious level. Intravenous fluid, at two-thirds normal maintenance, as dextrose–saline will optimize potentially compromised cerebral metabolism, will help avoid acidosis in the presence of an inborn error, and will prevent hypoglycaemia in Reye's syndrome. Other supportive care to maintain blood pressure and urine output and treat seizures and pyrexia will be necessary. If a cerebral tumour or bleed are identified, dexamethasone may help reduce surrounding oedema.

Answer 14.3

1. Guillain-Barré syndrome

Reject: Poliomyelitis

2. Nerve condition studies
   Electromyography

Discussion

Guillain-Barré syndrome is the commonest peripheral neuropathy in childhood. The main features are acute weakness, which is bilateral and symmetrical. Paraesthesia may be present. The paralysis is flaccid, with either adjacent or extremely reduced reflexes, the plantars being flexor. There may be loss of joint postural and superficial sensation, resulting in unsteadiness and impaired coordination, mimicking cerebellar ataxia. CSF findings may vary during the course of the disease, the rise in protein occurring up to 25 days after the onset in one study. Motor nerve conduction velocity is <70% of the lower limit in at least two nerves. A small proportion of cases may have evidence of axonal degeneration in addition to demyelination, and it has been suggested that in these cases the prognosis for complete recovery is worse. The finding of campylobacter in the stools is probably coincidental and not causally related to the development of Guillain-Barré syndrome.

Other causes of acute generalized weakness may be broadly classified as infectious (infectious myositis, enteroviral infection); metabolic (acute intermittent porphyria, tyrosinaemia); neuromuscular blockade (botulism, tick paralysis); and periodic paralysis. Muscular tenderness may be the presenting feature of poliomyelitis, but involvement is not symmetrical and there are no paraesthesia. Complete immunization makes the diagnosis less likely but does not exclude it. Asymmetrical weakness is often found in polymyositis, the reflexes frequently being preserved and bulbar lesions rare. Acute intermittent porphyria is rare in childhood, but its commonest presentation is a symmetrical muscular weakness often preceded by muscular pain or stiffness. It may rarely present with paraesthesia and urinary hesitency or retention. The tendon reflexes are absent or markedly reduced.

Answer 14.4

1. Pubertal gynaecomastia

2. Spontaneous resolution

3. Klinefelter's syndrome (47 XXY)
Hypogonadism
Hepatic tumours or cirrhosis
Thyroid disease
Testicular tumours
Adrenal tumours
Starvation
Drug, e.g. corticosteroids, ketoconazole, isoniazid, insulin, digitalis,
　　cimetidine, spironolactone, cytotoxic agents
Hyperprolactonaemia

Discussion

Pubertal gynaecomastia is common in teenage boys, typically beginning in Tanner stage 2 or 3 and lasting for up to 2 years. It has its peak prevalence between the ages of 12 and 15 years. Boys of this age often become aware of breast masses because they can be exquisitely tender. On examination unilateral or bilateral breast tissue may be localized under the areola (Type 1 gynaecomastia) or extending beyond the areola (Type 2 gynaecomastia).

Breast tissue will grow whenever the ratio of oestrogen to androgens is increased relative to normal adult male values. In early puberty, when increased oestrogens are secreted before the surging masculinizing hormones, ideal conditions exist for gynaecomastia to develop. The vast majority of adolescent gynaecomastia cases are due to this physiological cause.

It has been suggested that laboratory evaluation for endocrine disorders and liver function are indicated in the following circumstances:

— Condition persisting for >2 years;
— Onset of gynaecomastia precedes pubertal development;
— Onset of gynaecomastia occurs after physical maturation has occurred.

Answer 14.5

1. Family history of sickle cell disease
Family history of renal failure
Family history of deafness
Family history of clotting disorder, e.g. von Willebrand's disease, haemophilia or Christmas disease
Family history of porphyria
Family history of renal calculi

2. Bag a sample of urine for microscopy and culture
Abdominal ultrasound, including renal ultrasound
Abdominal X-ray
Clotting studies
Haemoglobin electrophoresis
Complement levels
ASOT titres

Cystoscopy

Discussion

A family history of deafness would suggest a diagnosis of Alport's syndrome, which is an X-linked recessive disorder in which males develop sensorineural deafness and end-stage renal failure in the late teens. Sickle cell disease may affect renal function and with acute crises gives rise to haemoglobinuria. This is not as likely as he is reported to be well at the time of the episodes of abnormally coloured urine. A disorder of haemostasis may also give rise to haematuria with acute episodes of bleeding. Vasculitides would reveal abnormal complement levels. Porphyria with acute exacerbation may also give rise to changes in urinary colour.

Microscopy is the most useful first-line investigation as it will differentiate haemoglobinuria from haematuria. It will also indicate the site of bleeding as the presence of dysmorphic red cells or casts are suggestive of parenchymal bleeding. Organisms and white cells in the urine are indicative of urinary tract infection; however, for this diagnosis to be made, a pure cultured growth of a single organism present at $>10^5$/ml is required. Abdominal ultrasound with abdominal X-ray are useful to identify obstruction, tumour or calculi. Clotting studies may indicate disorders of haemostasis. As a result, minor trauma may give rise to bleeding. Haemoglobin electrophoresis may confirm sickle cell disease. IgA deficiency and rheumatic fever are also associated with haematuria. Cystoscopy would probably be performed as a second-line investigation.

Paper 15 *QUESTIONS*

Question 15.1

A 3-week-old female infant was admitted having been found blue and not breathing at home. The child had seemed perfectly well prior to this incident and had taken a normal feed 2 h before. On finding the baby the mother had removed a small amount of vomit from the child's mouth and then started mouth-to-mouth resuscitation. The child responded almost at once and had then been brought to hospital by 999 ambulance.

The baby was the product of a normal pregnancy and weighed 4.1 kg at birth (39-weeks gestation). There had been no medical problems since birth. She was breast fed and was described as a greedy baby who often regurgitated a small amount of her feeds.

On examination she appeared to have made a full recovery. She was well cared for and well nourished, weighing 5.1 kg.

Full blood count	Normal
Serum urea and electrolytes	Normal
Full infection screen	Normal
Chest X-ray	Normal
ECG	Normal
EEG	Normal
Metabolic screen	Normal

2 days later a further apnoeic attack occurred in hospital whilst the baby was being bathed by a nurse. The child was due a feed and was not observed to vomit prior to the incident.

1. What is the diagnosis?
2. How would you confirm the diagnosis?
3. Would you discharge this infant with an apnoea alarm on medical grounds?

Question 15.2

A 3-month-old boy, the first of dizygotic twins, presented with acute pneumonia. He deteriorated and required mechanical ventilation. Following broncho-pulmonary lavage, *Pneumocystis carinii* was identified and subsequently his HIV antibody test was positive. His sister was healthy.

1. What is the risk of his twin sister having HIV infection?
2. How would you manage her now?

Question 15.3

A 6-year-old girl was referred for assessment of seizures refractory to treatment. She was born at term (birthweight 4.1 kg) after an uneventful pregnancy and delivery. Her parents were healthy and unrelated and she had a 10-year-old brother who was well. In the past, her walking was slightly delayed (24 months) and she was still using single words only at $3\frac{1}{2}$ years of age. At the age of 5 years she had had two episodes of sudden pallor and unresponsiveness associated with nystagmus and jerking of her right arm. These had settled spontaneously and an EEG had been reported as showing no focal epileptiform activity. She had been admitted to her local hospital in status epilepticus and her seizures had been difficult to control, despite maximum doses of several anticonvulsants singly and in combination over a period of several weeks. Partial control had finally been achieved using high doses of ACTH.

On examination she was Cushingoid and irritable. She was normotensive and there were no cranial bruits. Her head circumference was on the 25th centile. She was extremely tremulous and uncoordinated, but ocular movements were normal and fundoscopy was unremarkable. There were no focal physical signs, but she continued to have seizures involving the right arm, associated with nystagmus.

Urea and electrolytes	Normal
Serum ammonia	Normal
Albumin	25 g/dl
Alanine transferase	490 IU/l
Urine metabolic screen	Normal
Autoantibodies	Normal
Brain MRI	Severe cerebral atrophy
EEG	Grossly abnormal with an excess of slow activity and a paucity of rhythmic activity
Visually evoked responses	Asymmetrical
Electroretinogram	Normal

1. Suggest a diagnosis.

Question 15.4

A 10-year-old girl presented to casualty in a semicomatose state. She was found at a friend's house having consumed a mixture of spirits and sherry. There was no history of ingesting other substances. Full blood count and urea and electrolytes were normal. A high blood alcohol level was confirmed.

Her conscious state varied from being semicomatose to aggressive.

Because of her disruptive behaviour she was placed in a side room on a medical ward overnight. She had previously been well, but was on treatment with an inhaled steroid and intermittent ß-2 agonist for moderately severe asthma. Two h after admission she was found moribund in bed with Cheyne–Stokes respiration and a small amount of vomitus on the bed close to her head; blood pressure was normal and pupils reactive to light. The nursing staff had been monitoring her at 30-min intervals, measuring blood pressure and doing neurological observations. She had remained asleep but was responsive to painful stimuli.

1. What two laboratory investigations would you have performed in addition to those taken when she first attended casualty?
2. How else would you have monitored this child following admission to hospital?
3. Give three possible causes of the profound deterioration in her health.

Question 15.5

An 8-year-old Asian boy presented with bleeding from the left ear. There was a 4-week history of a serous-bloody discharge from this ear and for the past 4 days he had had severe pain in the ear. The GP prescribed gentamicin ear drops the week before but these had had no effect. There was no history of trauma and he said his hearing had not altered. He could still play games and had not had any episodes of abnormal gait.

There was nothing of note in his past medical history and he was fully immunized. He had not travelled outside the UK. He was born at full term by vaginal delivery weighing 6 lbs 7 ounces. He was an only child; his mother was a 33-year-old domestic supervisor at the hospital and his father a 35-year-old heavy goods vehicle driver.

On examination his height and weight were on the 50th centile and he was apyrexial. His gait was normal, he had no nystagmus and his general examination was otherwise normal. His right tympanic membrane was clearly seen and appeared normal. The left tympanic membrane was not clearly seen as there was an oval polyp obscuring the view. The polyp was friable and had surface ulceration, being about half the diameter of the external auditory canal. There were multiple bleeding points on the surface of the polyp. His throat, nose and mastoids were normal on examination. There was no lymphadenopathy. Weber testing was directed towards the right and the Rinne test was negative on the right and positive on the left.

1. What two investigations are required?
2. Give two possible diagnoses.

Paper 15 ANSWERS

Answer 15.1

1. Gastro-oesophageal reflux
'H'-type tracheo-oesophageal fistula

2. pH probe (alone or in combination with respiratory monitoring)

Barium study

Milk scan
Oesophagoscopy

3. No

Discussion

This child had gastro-oesophageal reflux. 'H'-type tracheo-oesophageal fistula whilst very rare (approx. 1 in 150 000 births) cannot be excluded. A history of frequent small vomits supports the diagnosis of gastro-oesophageal reflux, however, such a history is not always present. It is not unusual for reflux to cause apnoea at times when vomit is not observed. Confirmation of the diagnosis is best made using a pH probe in the lower oesophagus, ideally in combination with respiratory monitoring. Barium studies (e.g. barium swallow) will show reflux in about 30%.

The parents of this child would have been frightened by events and in such circumstances many would seek the 'reassurance' of an apnoea alarm. It is important to appreciate that the common respiratory monitoring systems are not reliable to detect obstructive episodes since they interpret the child's struggles to breathe as normal breaths. Whilst on medical grounds alone it is difficult to justify the use of an alarm, many parents do obtain alarms under these circumstances. If this is the case, it is essential that the family are taught infant resuscitation.

Answer 15.2

1. Less than the infected boy (i.e. <14% in the UK)

2. HIV-antibody status, together with:
— virus culture
— polymerase chain reaction for virus antigen
— P24 antigen
High dose cotrimoxazole (if virus status unknown or indeterminate)
Prophylaxis against pneumocystis (if virus status unknown or indeterminate)

Repeat HIV antibody at 18–24 months if virus status has yet to be determined

Reject: Any answer that does not cover the risks as given above
HIV-antibody tests without including antigen testing AZT as prophylaxis

Discussion

In the UK the risk of vertical transmission is approximately 14%. There is evidence based on twin studies that the second twin has a significantly lower risk, although a precise figure has not been determined.

The twin sister will have a positive HIV-antibody test but this is not sufficient to determine if she is infected by the virus as the majority of positive HIV tests in babies will be due to passively transferred maternal HIV antibodies. It is important therefore to proceed to indicators of virus infection, such as virus culture, polymerase chain reaction or P24 antigen identification. If any of these tests is positive this is conclusive evidence of infection. However, a negative result does not exclude the possibility of virus infection. In this situation it is normal to repeat the HIV-antibody test at 18 months by which time any passively transferred antibodies from the mother will have cleared from the circulation and a persisting HIV-antibody test will indicate true infection of the infant. Management also includes prophylaxis against *Pneumocystis carinii* pneumonia and currently cotrimoxazole is indicated for those children known to be infected. Treatment of babies with indeterminate status is controversial, although many centres recommend cotrimoxazole treatment until it is clear whether the infant has been infected or not. Current evidence suggests that prophylactic AZT (Zidovudine) is not indicated in children who are HIV positive but do not yet have the symptoms of AIDS.

Answer 15.3

1. Degenerative brain disease
Alper's disease (progressive neuronal degeneration of childhood)

Discussion

The normal EEG with an asymmetrical visual evoked response suggests asymmetrical involvement of the cerebral hemispheres in the disease process. The diagnosis of Alper's disease is supported by the electrophysiological findings and the grossly abnormal liver enzymes. It is uncertain whether it is a single entity or a group of disorders. It is usually inherited in an autosomal recessive fashion. The clinical picture varies with symptoms usually developing towards the end of the first year, although onset may be later in childhood. Fits are usually prominent and may be myoclonic or of the salaam type. Severe and progressive mental retardation with opisthotonus, spastic quadriplegia and deafness is the complete clinical picture, but in some cases ataxia and extrapyramidal rigidity may be the predominant clinical findings. Death usually occurs as a result of intractable seizures or liver failure. Definitive diagnosis can only be made by examination of brain tissue.

Answer 15.4

1. Blood glucose
   Toxicology screen

   Blood culture
   Blood gas
   CT scan
   Viral titres

   Liver function test

2. Admit to high-dependency unit (i.e. arrange for continuous observation)
   Regular blood glucose measurements
   Monitor ventilation

   Pass nasogastric tube

   Give antibiotics
   Give acyclovir

3. Vomiting with aspiration
   Profound hypoglycaemia
   Respiratory depression secondary to alcohol

   Progression of encephalopathy unrelated to alcohol
   Bleed into pre-existing cerebral tumour
   Unnoticed head injury

Discussion

A toxicology screen should be considered for all children presenting with confusion or coma even if, as in this case, the history suggests alcohol abuse.

Severe hypoglycaemia may accompany alcohol intoxication due to inhibition of glucogenesis. This occurs more commonly in children than adults. Typically, alcohol-induced hypoglycaemia occurs within 6–36 h of ingestion of a moderate to large amount of alcohol. Patients may lapse into coma and become hypothermic. The usual features of hypoglycaemia such as flushing, sweating and tachycardia are frequently absent.

Alcohol acts as a central nervous system depressant which in small doses interferes with cortical function, but which in large doses may depress medullary processes. The fatal dose of alcohol ingestion in children is difficult to estimate.

It is important to consider that pre-existing cerebral pathology may have affected this girl's behaviour and led to alcohol ingestion.

Answer 15.5

1. Cranial CT focusing particularly on the external and internal meatuses
Biopsy of polyp
Mantoux 1:10 000
Audiogram

2. Histiocytosis X
Rhabdomyosarcoma

Tuberculosis

Reject: Cholestatoma
Infected neurofibromata

Discussion

The lesion is friable and ulcerated, with surface bleeding points. These features raise the suspicion of a malignant lesion. The extent of the involvement is best determined by CT which will also help in planning exploratory surgery. Excision biopsy of this lesion will help to confirm the presence of malignancy, but specimens should be sent for culture, in particular for tuberculosis. Polyps are uncommon in the external auditory meatus and the two commonest malignancies in this area are histiocytosis X and rhabdomyosarcoma.

Cholestatoma will tend to impair hearing but does not have the appearance of a polyp. Neurofibromata is rejected as an answer as there is no evidence of axillary freckling, no café au lait patches, and no other neurofibromata.

Paper 16 *QUESTIONS*

Question 16.1

An 18-month-old female infant with Down syndrome returned for outpatient review. The child had been followed up from birth because of both Down syndrome and a complete atrioventricular canal defect which had been successfully treated with surgery at the age of 15 months.

Throughout her life the child had suffered with severe constipation. This took the form of very infrequent (weekly at best) bowel actions which were passed with great difficulty. Treatment in the form of lactulose and senna had not been helpful, however glycerine suppositories and micro-enemas did normally produce a bowel action.

Apart from the Down syndrome the child's perinatal history had been unremarkable. Prior to heart surgery general health had been relatively poor with frequent chest infections and a requirement for diuretics. This was the first child in the family and there was a younger brother of 6 weeks who was normal. Both parents were well with no history of constipation. The mother was a midwife and the father a clerical officer with a small company.

On examination the child appeared very well with good growth since her operation. Pulse rate was 96 beats/min and blood pressure 85/55 mmHg. She showed no signs of heart failure although she did have a residual murmur. In the abdomen there was some mild distension with one or two faecal masses easily palpable through lax abdominal musculature. Developmentally she showed some evidence of delay.

1. Suggest two possible diagnoses.
2. Give two investigations you would perform.

Question 16.2

A $2\frac{1}{2}$-year-old boy of Nigerian parents, who had recently visited Nigeria for the first time, presented with a 5-day history of fever, poor appetite and sleepiness. He had vomited on several occasions on the 2 days prior to admission and had also had several rigors in association with fever. On the day before admission he had stopped talking. The mother found him at 1.00 am on the night of admission lying in bed staring with his arms and legs rigid. When touched he pushed her away but was not vocalizing.

On admission he showed decerebrate posturing with fixed mid-point pupils and increased reflexes with equivocal plantar responses. His temperature was 38.2°C. There was no papilloedema, his gag reflex was depressed, there were no oculocephalic or oculovestibular responses, and there was no eye opening or limb withdrawal. His other vital signs were normal and his oxygen saturation was 94% in air. The past medical history was unremarkable. His CT scan was normal. A malaria film showed 25% parasitaemia.

1. What is the diagnosis?
2. What three therapeutic steps would you take?
3. What is the initial Glasgow coma score?
4. What is the likely outcome?

Question 16.3

A 4-week-old caucasian male infant was admitted following an episode of apnoea and cyanosis. He was born at term (birthweight 3.3 kg) after an uneventful pregnancy and delivery, being the second child of healthy parents. He had been breast fed and there had been no concerns until the brief apnoeic episode which had led to admission, although his mother felt that over the previous 12 h he had seemed quieter than usual.

Examination revealed a pale, hypotonic, lethargic baby. He was mildly jaundiced and the liver edge was palpable 1 cm below the costal margin. A presumptive diagnosis of septicaemia was made and full infection screen was performed. A lumbar puncture yielded a uniformly blood-stained cerebrospinal fluid and was therefore repeated, with the same result. A cranial ultrasound scan revealed bilateral intraventricular haemorrhage with mild ventricular dilatation. The infant had received 1 mg vitamin K i.m. at birth.

INR	1.8
Partial thromboplastin time with kaolin	54/43
Thrombin clotting time	25/15
Bilirubin	75 µmol/l (3–20 µmol/l)
Alanine transferase	97 IU/l (normal 2–53 IU/l)
Alkaline phosphatase	339 IU/l (normal <350 IU/l)
α-1-antitrypsin phenotype	ZZ

1. Suggest a possible cause for the intracranial haemorrhage.

Question 16.4

A 12-year-old boy presented following a 1-month history of cough. He had been seen by his GP and prescribed a ß2 agonist and oral penicillin. Ten days after treatment started he was sent to casualty following an episode of haemoptysis. There was a strong family history of asthma, hayfever and eczema. At the age of 4 years he had been treated with a bronchodilator for episodes of wheeze associated with upper respiratory tract infections. He lived with both parents and two older brothers. The family ran a boarding kennels.

When seen in hospital with this more recent illness, he was coughing up blood and a large amount of watery, slightly blood-stained fluid. He was noted to be mildly dyspnoeic with a respiratory rate of 30 breaths/min and he was apyrexial. No cutaneous abnormalities or rash were seen.

Haemoglobin	9 g/dl
White cell count	$13 \times 10^9/l$
Platelet count	$300 \times 10^9/l$
Blood film	Eosinophilia
Matoux test 1 in 1000	3.5 mm erythematous area at 48 h

1. What is the most likely diagnosis?
2. What two investigations would help you confirm your diagnosis?

Question 16.5

A boy was given 30 cubes of 1 inch size. These were coloured red, blue, green, yellow and orange; there were six cubes of each colour.

He could copy this bridge of three cubes.

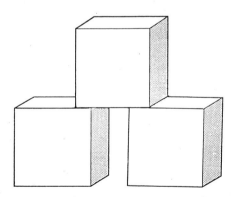

He was then asked to build a tower of red cubes. He did so making a tower of 6 cubes.

The examiner made three steps from six cubes without the boy having seen how to do this. The boy produced the shape shown overleaf.

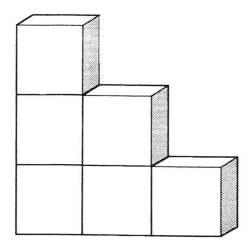

He was then asked to copy a circle, a cross, a square and a triangle and produced the following shapes:

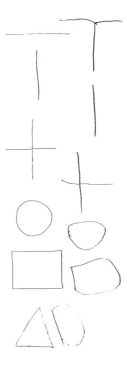

Then he was asked to draw a picture of a man and himself. He drew these figures.

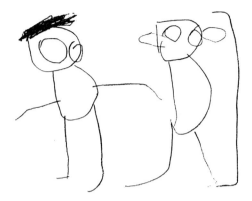

1. What is his developmental age?

PAPER 16 *ANSWERS*

Paper 16.1

1. Constipation secondary to Down syndrome
Hirschprung's disease (short-segment or ultra-short segment)

Hypothyroidism

2. Barium enema
Suction biopsy of the rectum
Thyroid function tests

Full thickness biopsy of the rectum
Rectal pressure studies

Discussion

Down syndrome is often complicated by constipation of some degree. Frequently this occurs in the absence of an anatomical or biochemical defect and is thought to result from a 'hypotonic' bowel. This can result in severe persistent constipation. Down syndrome is also associated with two other causes of constipation: hypothyroidism and Hirschprung's disease. In this child with normal pulse rate and relatively good developmental progress, hypothyroidism seems unlikely. However, it should be excluded both in this situation and where developmental progress is particularly poor, with or without constipation. Here long-segment Hirschprung's disease is not a possibility since it would have caused complete obstruction early in life. Short-segment disease may present in this way and is diagnosed reliably with suction biopsy, a simple outpatient procedure. Ultra-short segment disease represents a disconnection of the bowel musculature from the internal anal sphincter and is diagnosed by full thickness rectal biopsy (including the internal anal sphincter) under general anaesthetic. Rectal manometry is an investigation confined to a few specialist centres but which can be very helpful in difficult cases.

Answer 16.2

1. Cerebral malaria

Reject: Any other cause for his coma

2. Intravenous quinine
   Exchange blood transfusion
   Intravenous glucose
   Intubation and ventilation
   Intravenous mannitol

   Anticonvulsants
   Antibiotics

Reject: Oral chloroquine or other antimalarials
          Any other answer that is not appropriate for malaria

3. Eye opening   1
   Best motor response   2
   Best verbal response   1
                         ____
                            4

4. The prognosis is good

Discussion

Cerebral malaria is the explanation for his coma given his very high parasitaemia. This is a known complication and is usually confined to children who have not previously developed immunity from past exposure. This boy had never before been away from Britain. The pathogenesis is not clearly understood but involves a microangiopathy with vascular plugging and anoxia and may lead to cerebral oedema, although this is unusual and may be a terminal event. There is no other possible answer which is explained by the information given.

   The important principles of treatment include intravenous quinine because of the urgent need for effective treatment and the possibility of chloroquine resistance. Exchange blood transfusion is indicated when the erythrocyte parasitaemia percentage is >20 and has been shown to be effective. Intubation and ventilation will be required because of the coma, reduced gag reflex and the possibility of raised intracranial pressure (despite his having a normal CT scan which may not always demonstrate cerebral oedema). Intravenous mannitol is controversial although it may help where cerebral oedema is present. Anticonvulsants and antibiotics (pending blood cultures) may be useful. However, these are less appropriate answers than the above and would earn fewer marks.

   The Glasgow coma scale has been derived to produce uniformity in the assessment of unconscious patients. There is a modified score appropriate for children of various ages. A Glasgow coma score of 15 is normal; a score of 4 shows a severe degree of coma.

Modified Glasgow coma scale

		Score	< 1 year	> 1 year
EYE OPENING		4	Spontaneously	Spontaneously
		3	To shout	To verbal command
		2	To pain	To pain
		1	No response	No response
BEST		6		Obeys commands
MOTOR		5	Localizes pain	Localizes pain
RESPONSE		4	Flexion withdrawal	Flexion withdrawal
		3	Flexion abnormal	Flexion abnormal
		2	Extension	Extension
		1	No response	No response

		0–23 months	2–5 years	> 5 years
	5	Smiles, coos	Appropriate words	Orientated and converses
BEST		cries appropriately	& phrases	
VERBAL	4	Cries inappropriately	Inappropriate words	Disoriented and converses
RE-	3	Inappropriate crying	Cries +/or screams	Inappropriate words
SPONSE		or screaming		
	2	Grunts	Grunts	Incomprehensible sounds
	1	No response	No response	No response

The prognosis for this child's condition is good although untreated cerebral malaria inevitably progresses to death. The absence of cerebral oedema is a good prognostic sign.

Answer 16.3

1. α-1-antitrypsin deficiency

   Non-accidental injury
   Septicaemia

Reject: Haemorrhagic disease of the newborn

Discussion

Liver disease as a result of α-1-antitrypsin deficiency usually presents as an acute hepatitis in the first 4 months of life with conjugated hyperbilirubinaemia. This may either follow on from neonatal physiological jaundice or develop subsequently. Up to 10% of infants present with a bleeding diathesis due to vitamin K malabsorption, which tends to occur at a later stage than in classical haemorrhagic disease of the newborn. Between 40% and 50% of infants have abnormal biochemical tests of liver function through the first decade of life, often with no clinical evidence of liver disease. Presentation in later life with cirrhosis without antecedent neonatal hepatitis may occur.

Since the condition is inherited (autosomal co-dominant), it is essential that other family members are screened and genetic counselling given. Serum levels of α-1-antitrypsin may be increased or decreased by associated diseases or drugs and are therefore unreliable for diagnosis. Septicaemia is not excluded by the data given, and child abuse always needs consideration.

Answer 16.4

1. Ruptured hydatid cyst
   Bronchiectasis
   Pulmonary haemosiderosis

   Aspergillosis

2. Chest X-ray
   Casoni test
   Hydatid complement fixation test
   Bronchoscopy
   Blood clotting profile

   Aspergillus precipitans

Discussion

Haemoptysis is uncommon in children. However, sputum of children with suppurative lung disease, e.g. bronchiectasis and cystic fibrosis, is frequently streaked with blood due to bleeding granulation tissue in the affected bronchi. Occasionally a brisk haemoptysis occurs. These symptoms are mainly seen in older children or adolescents with well established disease. In this patient there is no history of chronic suppurative lung disease, making this unlikely.

Pulmonary haemosiderosis must be considered. The absence of telangiectatic skin lesions makes hereditary haemorrhagic telangiectasia unlikely. Primary tuberculosis infection rarely causes haemoptysis and in this case the Mantoux test is negative. With the child actually coughing up blood, but also coughing up watery blood-stained fluid followed by dyspnoea, a ruptured hydatid cyst is one of the most likely differential diagnoses. This is supported by the eosinophilia which is present in 70% of affected patients. The absence of temperature and lack of chronic symptoms make pulmonary infection and pulmonary vasculitis unlikely. Coagulopathy rarely causes haemoptysis.

Chest X-ray is essential and this may reveal segmental or lobar collapse, suggesting foreign body or, as in this case, a ruptured hydatid cyst. The cysts are usually round, uniformly opaque masses. However, following rupture, as in this case, the cysts appear as a rounded air-filled cavity with fluid level.

The Casoni test is performed by giving a 0.2 ml intradermal injection of sterile hydatid cyst fluid. A positive test is shown by a wheel of not <2 cm with a surrounding flare of >1 cm. The reaction develops within 30 min of injection. It is positive in approximately two-thirds of patients with hydatid cyst, but false positives can occur. The hydatid complement fixation test is more reliable than the Casoni test. A bronchoscopy is indicated in almost all patients presenting with haemoptysis. Clotting studies may be performed, though coagulopathy as a cause of haemoptysis is rare.

Answer 16.5

1. 4–5$\frac{1}{2}$ years

Discussion

A tower of three cubes can be built by most children at 18 months and up to eight cubes by the age of 2–2$\frac{1}{2}$ years. Larger towers are less discriminating.

Bridge building with three cubes can be imitated by most children at around 2 years 9 months of age. Making the three steps from six cubes without prior instruction tends to be performed by 5 years of age.

By 4 years of age children should recognize colours and can pick three out of four colours correctly. At 5 years of age 90% of children are able to distinguish colour.

The normal range for copying a circle is 2$\frac{1}{4}$–3$\frac{1}{2}$ years, a cross at 3–4$\frac{1}{2}$ years and a square by 4–5$\frac{1}{2}$ years. The triangle can be copied by the majority of children by 5$\frac{1}{2}$–6 years of age. It is important to note that these shapes are already drawn so that children are not merely able to imitate the examiner's efforts.

The Goodenough–Harris scoring system is applied to drawings of figures. This test has a detailed scoring system. One point is given for each of the following:

1 Head
2 Neck
3 Neck, two dimensions
4 Eyes
5 Eyebrows or eye lashes
6 Pupils of eyes
7 Nose
8 Nose in two dimensions
9 Mouth
10 Lips in two dimensions
11 Nose and lips in two dimensions
12 Chin and forebrow
13 Bridge of nose
14 Hair (any mess!)
15 Hair in greater detail
16 Ears
17 Fingers
18 Five fingers
19 Thumb opposed
20 Hands
21 Arms
22 Arms at side or involved in activity
23 Feet
24 Attachment of arms and/or legs to trunk anywhere
25 As in 24 but in correct position
26 Trunk
27 Trunk in proportion to body
28 Clothes — any
29 Two or more pieces of clothing

Draw-a-man

Age (years)	Score in boys
3	4
4	7
5	11
6	13
7	16
8	18

Girls tend to score higher in drawing than age-matched boys. The test also comprises drawing a figure of a woman which has a slightly different scoring system to include 'feminine shoes and neckline'.

Paper 17 *QUESTIONS*

Question 17.1

A 14-year-old boy presented acutely with a severe asthma attack which required intravenous steroids, frequent nebulized bronchodilators and oxygen over a number of days. He had been a severe asthmatic throughout his life. His maintenance therapy was inhaled steroid 1200 µg/day, inhaled bronchodilator and at times periods of alternate day oral steroids. He had been admitted over 50 times with acute attacks and had required ventilation on eight occasions. As well as hospital review his treatment was supervised by a private physician, a GP near his boarding school and a GP near his home. He was an only child. His parents were both well but divorced some years previously and were both remarried. The boy spent time with both parents but during school holidays was usually with his mother. Neither parent had a history of asthma. His father was 5ft 6in and his mother 5ft 4in.

At the time of discharge he was well with only mild residual wheeze and a normal peak flow. Pictures of his chest and his growth chart are shown overleaf. Previous growth hormone stimulation tests were normal.

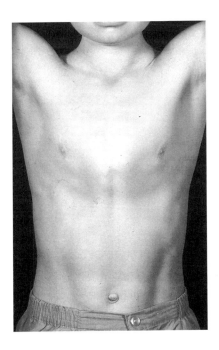 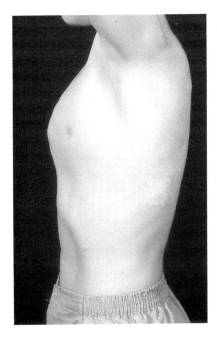

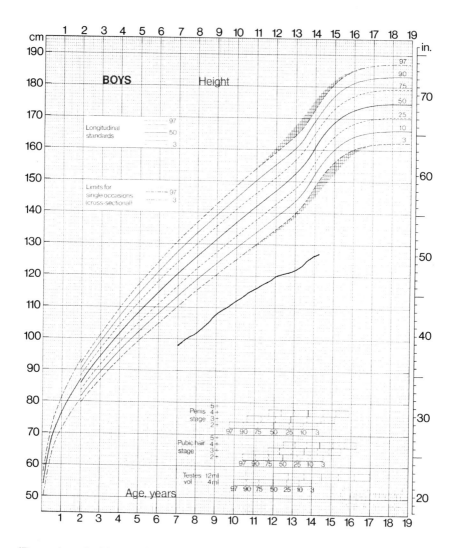

(Reproduced with permission of Castlemead Publications)

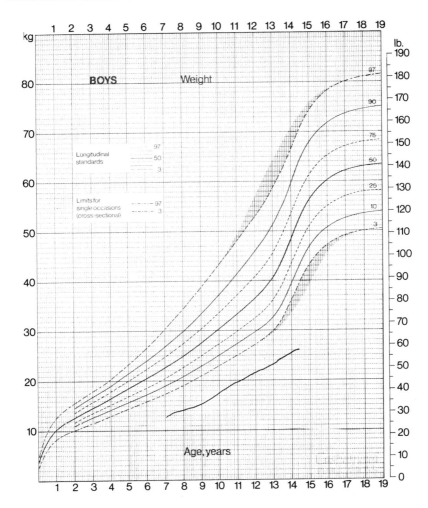

(Reproduced with permission of Castlemead Publications)

1. Describe the abnormality seen in the clinical picture.
2. Give the mechanism of the abnormalities noted in this picture.
3. Give three reasons for the boy's observed pattern of growth.
4. What is the prognosis regarding his final height?

Question 17.2

A $2\frac{1}{2}$-year-old caucasian boy was referred with a 1-month history of a slowly enlarging swelling in the left submandibular area. He was well, without generalized symptoms and the gland was only slightly uncomfortable. There had been no discharge. There had been no other illnesses in the preceding months and the family was well.

On examination there was a firm, mobile 2 cm diameter node with slightly purple discoloration of the overlying skin. It was slightly tender. Examination of the ears and throat was normal, there was no hepatosplenomegaly and there was no generalized lymphadenopathy.

Haemoglobin	12.2 g/dl
White cell count	$8.7 \times 10^9/l$
Lymphocytes	60%
Neutrophils	40%
Platelet count	$297 \times 10^9/l$
Chest X-ray	Normal

1. What is the most likely diagnosis?
2. How would you prove it?
3. How would you treat this particular case?

Question 17.3

A 9-year-old boy presented with a 3-day history of jaundice, nausea and anorexia. There had been no associated fever. His stools had been normal in colour but his urine was dark. On further questioning it became apparent that he had been slightly 'off colour' for the preceding 2 months and his school performance had deteriorated. In the past he had had pertussis at the age of 3 years and Henoch-Schönlein purpura at the age of 5 years. There was no history of contact with illness and he had been on no medication. He had a sister aged 7 years who was well.

On examination he was apyrexial, pale and mildly jaundiced. There were no cutaneous stigmata of chronic liver disease, but a firm, non-tender liver was palpable 5 cm below the costal margin. The spleen was also palpable 3 cm below the costal margin.

Haemoglobin	6.4 g/dl
White cell count	$5.2 \times 10^9/l$
Platelet count	$153 \times 10^9/l$
INR	1.9
Direct Coomb's test	Negative
Blood film	Absolute reticulocytosis, no evidence of recent haemolysis
Hepatitis A IgM	Negative
Hepatitis B serology	Negative
Paul-Bunnell test	Negative
Total protein	69 g/l
Albumin	29 g/l
Alkaline phosphatase	373 IU/l (normal <350 IU/l)

Gamma glutamyl transferase	63 IU/l (normal 5–55 IU/l)	
Alanine transferase	113 IU/l (normal 2–53 IU/l)	
Total bilirubin	33 µmol/l (normal 3–20 µmol/l)	
Abdominal ultrasound	Hepatosplenomegaly, solitary gallstone in gall bladder	

Urinalysis:

Glucose	++	
Reducing substances	1 g/l	
Amino acid screen	Concentration (µmol/mol creatinine)	Max. value (µmol/mol creatinine)
Threonine	336	46
Serine	371	97
Glycine	1293	617
Alanine	317	78
Tyrosine	115	16
Phenylalanine	37	15
Histidine	322	299
Ornithine	25	10
Lysine	139	30
Arginine	34	10

1. Suggest a possible diagnosis.
2. What three investigations would you perform next?

Question 17.4

A 5-month-old boy was admitted with a 5-day history of fever, vomiting and lethargy. In addition, his parents had noticed that he was generally much less active. The child was previously well with normal development. He had been bottle fed from birth and had had all his immunizations at the correct time.

On examination he was irritable and dyspnoeic. Blood pressure was raised at 120/70 mmHg. All limbs appeared flaccid but this was most marked in the right leg. Tendon reflexes could not be elicited. Facial muscles appeared paralysed bilaterally and ultrasound screening of the diaphragm showed the right dome to be paralysed. Peripheral sensation appeared normal.

Haemoglobin	12 g/dl
White cell count	14×10^9/el
C-reactive protein	1 mg/dl
EEG	Normal
EMG	Normal
Nerve conduction	44 m/s motor conduction in the left common peroneal, with a distal latency of 3 m/s (normal). 36 m/s (normal) sensory conduction in the right median nerve
CSF	39 polymorphonuclear cells/ml
Protein	0.5 g/l
Glucose	3 mmol/l
Blood glucose	4 mmol/l
Coxsackie B	Negative
Enterovirus	Negative

CSF 1 week later showed 37 white cells/μl, 34 of which were lymphocytes; protein 0.6 g/l; glucose 2.9 mmol/l. EMG was repeated 3 months later in the right quandriceps and tibialis anterior. Spontaneous activity, fibrillation and sharp waves were seen in both muscles, particularly in the lower part of the limb.

1. What further investigation would you perform?
2. What is the most likely diagnosis?
3. What immediate treatment would you have instigated on finding the initial CSF?

Question 17.5

A 2-year-old boy was well until 6 weeks ago when he developed central cramping abdominal pain, and his appetite started to decline. His parents noted that over the following 2 weeks he lost weight and became pale and lethargic. He had his bowels open daily and there was no change in his frequency of micturition. His parents took him to the GP who noted his general apathy and found the child had abdominal distension with diffuse tenderness. His liver was palpable to 4 cm below the right costal margin.

He was born by normal delivery weighing 6 lb without any subsequent neonatal problems. He had had no previous hospital admissions and was up to date with his immunizations. His mother worked in a bank and his father was a semi-professional football player. There was no family history of note.

On examination he was pale and had a distended abdomen. There was no lymphadenopathy. There was a mass of 10 cm × 5 cm below his left costal margin. His spleen was impalpable but his liver was 6 cm enlarged. There was genaralized tenderness over the abdomen but no bruit on auscultation. Normal bowel sounds were present. Cardiovascular examination revealed a regular pulse of 110 beats/min and blood pressure in the right arm of 150/90 mmHg. There were normal heart sounds with no murmurs. The respiratory system was clear with a respiratory rate of 10 breaths/min and the central nervous system examination was unremarkable.

Haemoglobin	7.4 g/dl
White cell count	10.2×10^9/l
Platelet count	312×10^9/l
Serum sodium	143 mmol/l
Serum potassium	3.9 mmol/l
Serum urea	5.2 mmol/l
Serum creatinine	35 mmol/l

1. Give three investigations which are required.
2. What is the diagnosis?

Paper 17 *ANSWERS*

Answer 17.1

1. Harrison's sulcus
Increased anteroposterior diameter

2. The Harrison's sulcus results from sustained overactivity of the diaphragm which deforms the chest. The increased anteroposterior diameter results from chronic overinflation, i.e. poorly controlled asthma

3. Chronic severe asthma

Constitutional short stature
Psychological/emotional factors
Chronic steroid use

4. He may reach a final height within 2 standard deviations of the mid parental height, because of the marked delay in bone age

Discussion

The boy has major problems with asthma. Both the history and the picture reveal clear evidence of recurrent and severe problems. The physical signs observed result jointly from chronic overactivity of respiratory muscles and persistent air trapping. The airways in this situation show sustained inflammatory changes.

The boy's short stature is a little more complex. There is no doubt that his asthma is sufficiently severe to cause impaired growth. In addition both parents are relatively small and this will have affected the boy's growth. The dose of inhaled steroids is at a level known to influence endogenous steroid production and he has also received further steroids by mouth. The use of excessive exogenous steroids may have contributed to the observed delay in bone age. The various psychological stresses that the boy has encountered must also be considered both in the context of the boy's severe asthma and in their own right.

Because of the marked delay in bone age the boy's period of growth may be extended and as a result allow him to achieve a final height within the normal range.

Answer 17.2

1. Atypical mycobacterial infection

Chronic lymphadenitis (non-specific)
Acute lymphadenitis
Malignancy, e.g. neuroblastoma, lymphoma, leukaemia
Tuberculosis

Branchial cyst
Submandibular calculus

Reject: Sternomastoid tumour
Lymphangioma

2. Biopsy for microscopy and culture
Mantoux testing with specific PPD for variety of atypical mycobacterial
organisms
Conventional Mantoux test
Chest X-ray

3. Surgical removal

Discussion

The most acceptable answer is a diagnosis of a non-tuberculous or atypical mycobacterial infection. Atypical mycobacterial infection is an increasingly recognized condition in an otherwise healthy child and is characterized by a slowly growing mass without evidence of an acute infection or inflammation. Chronic or acute-on-chronic lymphadenitis is much less likely given the absence of acute signs. The blood count is inconsistent with acute infection or malignancy but it does not completely exclude these diagnoses. Mycobacterium tuberculosis only very rarely presents in this way, particularly without other signs. Other rare possibilities which are much less acceptable answers are a cyst or a calculus.

Ideally, such infection is identified by surgical removal followed by microscopy and culture. This is also the treatment of choice as well as providing a diagnosis. Other conditions in the differential diagnosis would be excluded on microscopy. Rarely, if surgical removal is not possible because of the site of the node, treatment with combination therapy including isoniazid, ciprofloxacin, cotrimoxazole and azithromycin may be useful. Conventional triple therapy for tuberculosis is inappropriate; these organisms are not sensitive. Surgical removal is also the appropriate answer for other surgical conditions while chemotherapy is indicated for leukaemia, lymphoma or other malignancies.

Answer 17.3

1. Wilson's disease

2. Serum caeruloplasmin
Slit-lamp examination of the eyes
Urinary copper excretion with penicillamine challenge
Liver biopsy for copper content
Investigate sibling

Reject: Serum copper level

Discussion

Any child presenting with an unexplained hepatic illness, general ill health or deteriorating school performance must have Wilson's disease considered as a possible diagnosis. More than 50% of cases present before puberty with no neurological abnormality. The disease is characterized by defective biliary copper excretion with high concentrations being found in the liver, brain, corneas and renal tubules of affected patients. The most constant biochemical abnormality found is a low serum concentration of caeruloplasmin, which transports copper. Very rapid copper release from damaged cells is thought to cause the haemolytic anaemia which may occur early in the disease, as in this case. Renal involvement may mimic nephrotic syndrome or present as renal rickets and a Fanconi syndrome.

A low serum caeruloplasmin is suggestive of Wilson's disease, although it may also be found in nephrotic syndrome, severe malabsorption or protein-losing enteropathy. Up to 20% of patients with Wilson's disease may however have normal caeruloplasmin levels. Slit-lamp examination of the eye may reveal Kayser–Fleisher rings as green/brown deposits of copper just within the limbus. Serum copper levels are not helpful in the diagnosis, but urinary copper excretion is increased, and rises further after penicillamine.

Since there may be no abnormalities on clinical examination, ophthalmic slit-lamp examination, hepatic and renal biochemistry, serum caeruloplasmin estimation and urinary copper determination (with and without penicillamine) need to be performed. If any of these are abnormal, the next step should be liver biopsy for copper determination.

Answer 17.4

1. Viral serology (especially polio)

   MRI or CT scan of head

2. Poliomyelitis

   Guillain-Barré syndrome

3. Intravenous broad-spectrum antibiotics
   Intravenous acyclovir

Discussion

The child had been immunized 1 month previously and this is a typical case of polio following vaccination. Virology for polio virus is thus essential. Ultrasound, CT and MRI scan are often indicated in patients with unusual neurological symptoms.

   Delayed appearance of nerve stimulation/EMG abnormalities are characteristic of both Guillain-Barré syndrome and poliomyelitis.

   A high white cell count in the initial CSF means an infective cause cannot be excluded. Therefore treatment with antibiotics and an antiviral agent (acyclovir), is indicated initially.

Answer 17.5

1. Urinary catecholamines
   Abdominal X-ray
   Ultrasound of abdomen
   Bone marrow biopsy
   MIBG (an isotope scan specific for chromaffin tissue)
   DTPA scan
   Chest X-ray
   Serum renin level
   Abdominal and chest CT

2. Neuroblastoma

   Wilm's tumour

   Rhabdomyosarcoma
   Phaeochromocytoma
   Polycystic kidney disease

Reject: Primary hypertension

Discussion

Neuroblastoma is the most likely diagnosis as there is weight loss, an abdominal mass and hypertension (due to catecholamine release). The enlargement of the liver is explained by the presence of secondaries.

Wilm's tumour and rhabdomyosarcoma are less likely to cause hypertension. Phaeochromocytomae are very rare in childhood and are associated with sudden release of catecholamines giving rise to episodic hypertension rather than consistently raised blood pressure. Polycystic kidney disease is unlikely to give this clinical picture, especially hepatic enlargement.

Paper 18 *QUESTIONS*

Question 18.1

A 42-week gestation male infant was born following a spontaneous onset of labour. The birth was uncomplicated. The midwife at the delivery was immediately concerned because of the unusual appearance of the child's skin (see picture). Apart from the skin abnormalities the child seemed well and no other anomalies were noted. He was the parent's first child and was conceived after a course of ovarian stimulation. Both parents were well and there was no family history of skin disorder.

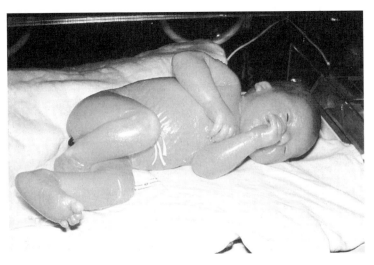

The child was admitted to the neonatal nursery for a period of observation. Bottle feeding was established without difficulty. His skin continued to crack and flake revealing an epidermis that was hyperaemic and which leaked serous fluid. On the third day of life the infant became lethargic and showed evidence of temperature instability.

Haemoglobin	20.2 g/dl
White cell count	$16.7 \times 10^9/l$
Platelet count	$234 \times 10^9/l$
Sodium	141 mmol/l
Potassium	5.8 mmol/l
Urea	8.6 mmol/l
HCO$_3$	18.4 mmol/l
Glucose	3.4 mmol/l
CSF glucose	1.2 mmol/l

CSF protein	0.4 g/l
CSF microscopy	100 red blood cells, 209 white blood cells, no organisms seen
Urine osmolality	500 mOsmol/kg

1. What is the condition seen in the picture?
2. What is the prognosis for the skin in this condition?
3. What is the likely explanation for the baby's illness at 3 days?

Question 18.2

A 13-year-old girl who had had acute lymphoblastic leukaemia treated over the past 3 years and was in her final maintenance therapy with methotrexate and vincristine, presented with a cough. She was asthmatic and used intermittent ß-agonist. She was not taking other medication and had been well until the past 4 weeks.

On examination she was wheezy and tachypnoeic, and had a temperature of 37.8°C. Her saturation in air was 90%, peak expiratory flow 250 l/min (normal 250–350 l/min) and her chest X-ray was hyperinflated but otherwise normal.

Blood gases (arterial):
pH	7.45
PaO_2	4.0 kPa
$PaCO_2$	9.0 kPa

1. What is the diagnosis?
2. How would you treat her?

Question 18.3

A 5-year-old boy was referred with a 1-week history of reduced use of his left arm and leg. His parents had also noticed that his coordination with the left arm was reduced, and he was tending to drop objects when held in that hand. They said that some of the movements of the arm were abnormal. He complained that his left leg felt 'heavy'. He had recently started at school and had not settled in well, being described by his teacher as rather restless (and hence disruptive) in class. Over the same period of time his parents felt that his behaviour had greatly deteriorated. The only past history of note was chickenpox 5 months ago. His older brother recently had presumed hepatitis A, which resolved quickly.

On examination he looked well, was apyrexial and was appropriately grown. He appeared fidgety and was unsteady on his feet. The power in his left leg and arm was reduced and he had poor finger–nose coordination. His reflexes were slightly reduced on the left side, but his plantar reflexes were down-going. Systemic examination was otherwise unremarkable and he was normotensive.

Haemoglobin	13.1 g/dl
White cell count	12.0×10^9/l
Platelet count	314×10^9/l
Serum electrolytes	Normal
CT head scan	No midline shift, no parenchymal abnormality seen
CSF	0 red cells, 0 white cells, protein 0.1 g/l, glucose 3.5 mmol/l

1. Suggest a possible diagnosis.
2. What further investigations would you perform?

Question 18.4

A male infant was born at 37 weeks gestation weighing 3.7 kg. He was the mother's second child, and her pregnancy was normal apart from chickenpox at 30 weeks gestation. Delivery was by caesarean section performed for a prolonged second-stage of labour. The infant developed mild respiratory distress which was diagnosed as transient tachypnoea of the newborn. A septic screen was performed, including a lumbar puncture which was normal, and the child commenced on penicilin and gentamicin. Within 24 h the child had recovered completely from his respiratory distress. On day 3, while still on the neonatal unit, he suffered a marked apnoeic episode. Blood glucose was 0.5 mmol/l. There had been no previously recorded low blood sugars. Following an intravenous bolus of glucose there was a dramatic improvement in his condition. An intravenous infusion of dextrose was continued to maintain the blood sugar at a normal level.

(following treatment of hypoglycaemia):

Haemoglobin	15 g/dl
White cell count	15×10^9/l
Serium calcium	2.3 mmol/l
Liver function tests	Normal
Arterial pH	7.35
$PaCO_2$	4.8 kPa
PaO_2	12 kPa
Lactate	1.6 mmol/l (normal 0.63–2.5 mmol/l)
Urine ketones	Negative
Plasma ammonia	Normal
Plasma and urinary amino acids	Normal

Glucose	2 mmol/l
Insulin	20 mU/l (high)
Growth hormone	20 mU/l
Cortisol	600 nmol/ml (normal 140–800 nmol/ml)

Several hours later the child became hypoglycaemic with a blood sugar of 0.8 mmol/l. At this stage, insulin was 35 mU/l (high).

1. What is the most likely diagnosis?
2. What other information may support your diagnosis?
3. The mother had a medical training and the father was diabetic. Munchausen-by-proxy was included in the differential diagnosis. How can you exclude this diagnosis?
4. What treatment may be required?

Question 18.5

A 16-year-old Asian boy was referred by an ENT consultant who had noted that the teenager had a productive cough and bilateral basal crackles and rhonchi on auscultation. He was initially referred by his GP as he had had recurrent bouts of frontal and maxillary pain which had not responded to several courses of antibiotics over a 3-month period.

He had returned from India about 3 years ago, having been born in the UK at term weighing 7 lbs. He moved to live with relatives in India when 6 years old. His past medical history was unremarkable. His immunizations were up to date including neonatal BCG immunization.

Sputum sent at this consultation was macroscopically thick and purulent but failed to grow any organisms.

Haemoglobin	12 g/dl
White cell count	10×10^9/l
Neutrophils	60%
Lymphocytes	38%
Monocytes	2%
Platelet count	243×10^{12}/l

The family reported that he had had some tests performed in India just prior to returning. They brought the investigation shown opposite to clinic.

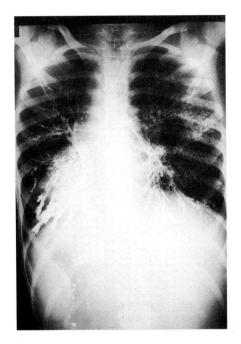

1. What is the investigation?
2. What abnormalities are seen?
3. What other investigation is warranted?

Paper 18 ANSWERS

Answer 18.1

1. Collodian baby

2. At this early stage it is not possible to give a prognosis since 'collodian' baby is not a diagnosis but a descriptive term. Some of the underlying pathological processes will resolve completely, whilst others will persist as severe ichthyosis throughout life

3. Vasomotor collapse
Sepsis/meningitis
Dehydration

Reject: Hypoglycaemia
Diabetes insipidus

Discussion

At the time the baby became overtly unwell he had developed two separate problems. As the skin flaked the underlying surface remained abnormal (some 'collodian' babies have skin which is entirely normal once the outer collodian layer is removed) and under these circumstances the baby was exposed both to enhanced fluid loss and increased infection risk. The results in this baby show evidence that both had occurred. There is no association between the various skin conditions that lead to 'collodian' babies and immune deficiency, however, the abnormal skin remains an easy portal of entry for infection and this infant in fact suffered a second episode of meningitis some weeks later.

The evidence of normal urine osmolarity precludes a diagnosis of diabetes insipidus.

Answer 18.2

1. *Pneumocystis carinii* pneumonia

Atypical pneumonia

Asthma
Interstitial pneumonitis
Reaction to vincristine
Bacterial pneumonia

2. Oxygen therapy
   Cotrimoxazole

   Erythromycin
   Steroids

   Increased ß-agonists
   Broad-spectrum antibiotics
   Artificial ventilation

Discussion

The important principle to consider is the potential for immunosuppression by methotrexate and vincristine. Her asthma may contribute to her respiratory symptoms but she is febrile, her peak flow is just at the lower end of the normal range, she is significantly hypoxic and hypercarbic and her chest X-ray shows no consolidation. The most likely explanation is an atypical pneumonia, *pneumocystis carinii* being the most probable in this situation. A mycoplasma might also produce these findings. Bacterial pneumonia is a much less likely possibility. Rarely methotrexate may produce an interstitial pneumonitis and vincristine may provoke persisting bronchospasm.

The management of *Pneumocystis carinii* pneumonia includes oxygen for hypoxia, high-dose intravenous or oral cotrimoxazole for 2 weeks and a concurrent course of steroids. An antibiotic, e.g. erythromycin, to cover mycoplasma would be useful pending indentification of the organisms, or if a bacterial pneumonia is diagnosed, broad-spectrum antibiotics are indicated. Increased nebulized ß-agonists are required to treat the asthmatic component of her symptoms. Rarely, mechanical ventilation is indicated for respiratory failure.

Answer 18.3

1. Unilateral chorea
   Sydenham's chorea
   Lupus-associated chorea
   Thyrotoxicosis

Reject: Behaviour disorder

2. Antistreptolysin O titre
   Antinuclear antibodies
   Thyroid function
   Echocardiogram

Discussion

Sydenham's chorea was the most common form of acquired chorea in children. Its incidence declined greatly but has begun to increase again. It is a major manifestation of rheumatic fever, which develops in one-third of untreated patients. Onset may be acute or insidious, and is much more common in girls. The onset may be several months after the initial streptococcal infection and therefore the antistreptolysin O titre may be normal. The major clinical features are chorea, hypotonia, normal reflexes and emotional lability; seizures are rare, but there may be abnormalities on EEG. The choreiform movements are of a high order and quasi-purposive. They always disappear during sleep. Bilateral facial movements may mimic emotional changes. The behavioural changes may be thought to be a sign of mental illness. The chorea is generalized in most patients, but may be unilateral ('hemichorea') in the early stages.

All children with Sydenham's chorea need to be treated as if they have acute rheumatic fever with high-dose penicillin to eradicate streptococcal infection, followed by prophylactic penicillin therapy until adulthood.

Diagnosis is essentially clinical although it is difficult to distinguish between Sydenham's and lupus-associated chorea. The latter may occur from 7 years before to 3 years after systemic manifestations of the disease. Approximately 25% of these patients have relapses of chorea, and following the appearance of systemic features neurological complications such as seizures, ataxia and psychosis are common. The finding of a raised antinuclear antibody titre is diagnostic.

Answer 18.4

1. Persistent neonatal hypoglycaemia due to nesidioblastosis

Infant of a diabetic mother (undiagnosed in mother)
Munchausen by proxy

Reject: Glycogen storage disease
Ketotic hypoglycaemia

2. Very high glucose infusion rates to maintain normoglycaemia
Elevation of plasma pancreatic polypeptide

3. C-peptide levels

Video/covert surveillance

4. Concentrated glucose infusions
Oral diazoxide
Glucagon
Intravenous somatostatin
Surgical pancreatectomy

Discussion

The most likely diagnosis is nesidioblastosis. In cases of nesidioblastosis the patient has hypoglycaemia but the insulin is inappropriately elevated. In addition there is no deficiency of counter regulatory hormones such as growth hormone and cortisol, lactate is normal and ß-hydroxybutyrate is normal or decreased. Nesidioblastosis refers to the structural disorganization of the endocrine pancreas with an excess of ß-cells. Infants often present with refractory hypoglycaemia, continuing beyond the neonatal period.

Munchausen-by-proxy syndrome should always be considered in patients with unusual symptoms. However, if C-peptide levels are normal this is unlikely. C-peptide is part of the connecting chain which remains intact during the conversion of proinsulin to insulin. It is secreted in equimolar amounts with insulin and is a useful marker of ß-cell function.

It is often impossible to keep pace with hypoglycaemia in patients with nesidioblastosis. This is despite a continuous dextrose infusion. In this child, a glucose infusion rate of 13 mg/kg/min was required while the normal is 6–8 mg/kg/min. Medical treatment includes glucose infusions, but hyperinsulinism may have to be controlled with oral diazoxide. This may fail and surgical pancreatectomy must be planned to avoid life-threatening hypoglycaemia. An intravenous infusion of somatostatin combined with glucagon may give time to plan surgery. At operation, approximately 80% of the pancreas is resected. Even so, some children will require a secondary operation to remove even more of the pancreatic remnant.

Answer 18.5

1. Bronchogram

2. Bronchiectasis
Dextro-cardia
Situs inversus

Reject: Increased shadowing
Aspiration
Pneumonia

3. Ciliary biopsy for motility studies

Mantoux 1:10 000 intradermal test
Sweat test
Immunoglobulin levels including IgG sub-class values
Ventilation–perfusion scan
Bronchoscopy

Discussion

The investigation shown is a bronchogram with bronchiectasis. It should also be noted that there is a dextro-cardia with situs inversus. The overall clinical picture suggests Kartegener's syndrome. Hence the most accurate answer for investigation is ciliary motility studies. Other causes of bronchiectasis include: tuberculosis, immunodeficiency including IgG_2 sub-class deficiency, measles, whooping cough, foreign body and cystic fibrosis.

Paper 19 *QUESTIONS*

Question 19.1

A 27-week-gestation girl was delivered by emergency caesarian section for fetal distress. Birth weight was 1.2 kg. There had been a spontaneous onset of labour, probably precipitated by polyhydramnios. The baby was in good condition at birth but developed respiratory distress. The baby received full intensive care support, including maintenance intravenous fluids, and soon stabilized. A septic screen was performed and broad-spectrum antibiotics commenced.

She was the second child in the family. The first had also been born prematurely and had died at the age of 10 months. That baby's course had been complicated by severe birth asphyxia, renal failure and mental retardation. The child's father was in the army and the mother a secretary. Both were well.

Towards the end of the second day of life the child became unwell with increasing core peripheral temperature gap, tachycardia and decreased movements. Blood glucose was normal and the child was noted to be passing urine in good amounts. The child's weight was 0.94 kg.

(at the time of deterioration)

Haemoglobin	23 g/dl	
White cell count	18.9×10^9/l	
Platelet count	345×10^9/l	
Sodium	148 mmol/l (blood)	36 mmol/l (urine)
Potassium	6.0 mmol/l (blood)	12 mmol/l (urine)
Urea	8.9 mmol/l (blood)	44 mmol/l (urine)
Osmolality	3.9 mOsmol/kg (blood)	357 mOsmol/kg (urine)
Capillary pH	7.31	
Initial blood cultures	Normal	

1. What is the cause of the child's severe electrolyte abnormalities?
2. Suggest two further investigations.
3. Suggest a diagnosis.

Question 19.2

A 2-year-old boy was seen in the Paediatric A&E department. His foster mother said she found him with an empty bottle which once contained drain cleaner, but which had been rinsed out with water. On examination he had blisters in his mouth and the front of his tongue but none was seen more posteriorly or in the pharynx. He was refusing to drink or eat but did not complain of pain other than around his lips.

1. What is the immediate management?

2. How would you manage the next 24 h?

Question 19.3

A 14-month-old girl presented with a 3-week history of increasing breathlessness. She was born at 36-weeks gestation, the first of twins. There were no neonatal problems. Her birthweight was on the 3rd centile and had increased appropriately. Her twin sister was well.

On examination she looked pale. Her respiratory rate was 55 breaths/min, with marked intercostal recession and Harrison's sulci. There were bilateral fine crackles on auscultation. Her pulse was 120 beats/min, heart sounds were normal, and there was a 3/6 systolic murmur heard best at the left lower sternal edge. There was no hepatomegaly.

Haemoglobin	7.7 g/dl
White cell count	$8.1 \times 10^9/l$
Platelet count	$229 \times 10^9/l$
MCV	74 fl
MCH	23 pg
Chest X-ray	Cardiomegaly, plethoric lung fields
Echocardiogram	Perimembranous ventricular septal defect
Cardiac catheter	Systemic pressure 100 mmHg, pulmonary artery pressure 45 mmHg, pulmonary: systemic blood flow 1.4:1

1. What is the cause for this child's symptoms?

2. How would you manage the case?

Question 19.4

An 11-year-old girl presented with a 3-week history of inflammation affecting both knees and one elbow. Initially her elbow was affected and became hot, red, tender and swollen. As this was improving, a similar problem developed in her left and then her right knee.

On examination she had a tachycardia, a temperature of 38.5°C and a systolic murmur radiating to the axilla was clearly heard. Her heart was thought to be normal on auscultation when admitted for appendicectomy at 8 years of age.

Over the next 3 days she developed an area of erythema over her body. Her chest was clear on auscultation and no abnormalities were found on abdominal examination.

Haemoglobin	13×10^9/l
White cell count	18×10^9/l
ESR	95
C-reactive protein	Raised

1. What is the most likely diagnosis?
2. Give two investigations that may be helpful in establishing the underlying diagnosis?

Question 19.5

A 16-year-old girl was seen in outpatients with a month's history of intermittent central abdominal pain and weight loss. Her appetite had declined over the same period and she felt generally unwell. Her bowels were open once a day with no change in consistency. She had not had any bouts of diarrhoea or bloody stools.

Her periods were regular. She was not taking any medications other than up to 1 g of paracetamol when the pain was at its worst. The bouts of pain could last all day and had woken her in the night. The pain was a dull continuous ache with occasional stabbing pains located at about the centre of the abdomen.

On examination there was nothing abnormal to find apart from the picture shown.

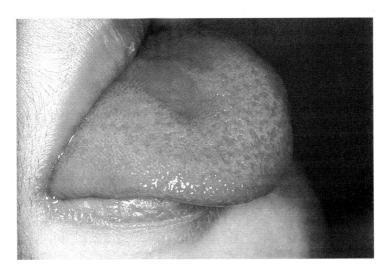

1. Describe the appearance of the abnormality seen.
2. Give the diagnosis.

Paper 19 *ANSWERS*

Answer 19.1

1. Dehydration

2. Renal ultrasound
Renal isotope scan (DTPA)
Urinary steroid profile
Urinary amino acids
Urinary protein
Urinary glucose
Urine pH
Careful fluid balance calculations

Karyotype
Plasma renin/angiotensin

3. Nephrogenic diabetes insipidus (secondary to immaturity)
Nephrogenic diabetes insipidus (primary)

Renal tubular defect

Discussion

This is a complex case. There is evidence that supports the presence of polyuria: the history of polyhydramnios, excessive weight loss over the first 2 days of life, continued good urine output in the face of dehydration. At 2 days the child has very clear evidence of dehydration.

The aim in assessing this child must be to try and determine whether there is evidence of structural renal anomaly, a tubular defect, or a hormonal abnormality. However, some aspects of the investigation of this baby are complicated by the child's immaturity. At 27-weeks gestation normal tubular function is not established and excessive renal electrolyte losses are relatively common. Similarly, urinary steroid excretion will reflect fetal pattern. The technical difficulties surrounding the estimation of renin and angiotensin make this a low priority.

The excessive renal fluid loss, normal pH and lack of evidence of a specific tubular defect of electrolyte homeostasis makes diabetes insipidus the most likely diagnosis. In reality the child's problems resolved completely at about 1 year of age.

Answer 19.2

1. Intravenous access and fluids (10–20 ml/kg) if indicated to establish

haemodynamic stability
Oxygen and mask or endotracheal tube if there is respiratory compromise
Chest X-ray
Intravenous fluid maintenance
Respiratory support if indicated

Reject: Nasogastric tube
Emetic
Prophylactic steroids
Prophylactic antibiotics
Neutralizing chemicals

2. Oesophagoscopy
Gastroscopy
Insertion of nasogastric tube after this procedure
Manage shock and respiratory distress as in answer 1 above
Antibiotics if infection develops
Nutritional support by nasogastric tube or intravenously
Emergency oesophagectomy with jejunostomy or gastrostomy if oesophageal damage is severe

Reject: Oral feeding (unless the patient is able to swallow)
Dilation of the oesophagus
Steroids

Discussion

The first question deals with the principles of resuscitation. Although the clinical findings might suggest that the caustic ingestion has damaged only the anterior part of the mouth, it is possible for the posterior pharynx not to have come into contact with the ingested material, but swallowing might still have carried the caustic material into the oesophagus. Some children may have cardiovascular and respiratory compromise when they present and it is essential in the answer to cover the principles of providing support. A nasogastric tube should not be passed until the oesophagus has been assessed under direct vision as perforation may occur.

There is no evidence for the use of prophylactic steroids or antibiotics. Emetics should not be in given as perforation or aspiration may occur, producing further damage by depositing corrosive material onto the epiglottis, vocal cords and larynx. Neutralizing chemicals will produce heat and may cause further damage. A chest X-ray is useful to diagnose pneumonitis or perforation.

The priority in subsequent management is to assess the severity of oesophageal involvement by endoscopy within 24–48 h. A nasogastric tube may then be passed for nutritional purposes and to maintain luminal patency. Even at this later stage there is no place for prophylactic steroids or antibiotics, although antibiotics are indicated for pneumonitis or mediastinitis.

Answer 19.3

1. Ventricular septal defect with anaemia

Reject: Ventricular septal defect
Anaemia

2. Treat anaemia and reassess

Reject: Close ventricular septal defect

Discussion

The child's ventricular septal defect is not haemodynamically significant enough to cause the clinical picture of pulmonary oedema, and an otherwise well child with a haemoglobin at this level will not present in this way. However, the combination of a shunt and anaemia will result in pulmonary oedema since the reduction in blood viscosity, caused by the anaemia, will produce increased pulmonary blood flow. This child's anaemia should be treated before further consideration is given to the ventricular septal defect.

Answer 19.4

1. Rheumatic fever

Subacute bacterial endocarditis
Innocent murmur with febrile illness (i.e. viral, mycoplasma)
Juvenile rheumatoid arthritis

Bacterial arthritis
Henoch–Schönlein purpura
Still's disease

2. Throat swab
Antistreptolysin-O titre (if low an antistreptococcal-antibody assay)
ECG
Two-dimensional echocardiography

Reject: Cardiac catheter

Discussion

The occurence of a significant heart murmur (mitral insufficiency), flitting arthritis and rash (Erythema marginatum) make the diagnosis of rheumatic fever very likely. The raised white cell count, C-reactive protein and ESR are supportive but seen in many of the other possible diagnoses listed. The murmur is obviously significant in this child and not a pulmonary flow murmur which is often heard in sick pyrexial children. Bacterial endocarditis should be strongly considered as it may cause cardiac damage accounting for new murmurs, athritis and rash. Occasionally a viral infection may cause myocarditis, rash and joint swelling. A very high C-reactive protein is not usually seen with viral infections alone.

It is essential to demonstrate recent streptococcal infection, usually by elevation of antistreptolysin-O titre. An ECG may show characteristic prolongation of the P–R and Q–T intervals. Second-degree, or even complete, atrioventricular block may occur due to inflammation of the conduction system. Two-dimensional echocardiography would confirm the clinical picture of mitral insufficiency in this patient.

The diagnosis of rheumatic fever is important because subsequent serious cardiac disease can be prevented or markedly reduced by long-term antistreptococcal treatment.

Answer 19.5

1. Two shallow based ulcers in the centre of the tongue and an ulcer on the upper lip margin

   Apthous ulcers

Reject: Geographical tongue

2. Crohn's disease

   Coeliac disease

Reject: Anorexia/bulaemia
Syphilis
Behcet's syndrome

Discussion

The history of abdominal pain, weight loss and ulcers is indicative of Crohn's disease. Ulcers such as snail-track ulcers of syphilis do not fit the case history. Behcet's disease occurs with perianal ulceration and arthropathy. It is rare in this age group.

Paper 20 QUESTIONS

Question 20.1

A 2-year-old boy presented to outpatients with a history of severe and persistent diarrhoea. The problem had first been noted at about 6 months of age and had seemed to get worse as the child became established on a more solid diet. At the time of referral the boy opened his bowels approximately 6–8 times/day. On each occasion he produced a watery stool. His mother was extremely distressed not only because of the persistent nature of the problem but also because of the mess the child caused. Her concern was increased by the fact that it was often possible to recognize items of food in the stools. Apart from this problem he was a well child who was developing normally.

The boy had an older brother who was well as were both parents. His father was a refuse collector and his mother a housewife. They lived in their own house which was centrally heated.

On examination the boy looked healthy and was cooperative. Apart from a minor protuberance of his abdomen, there were no abnormalities. His growth chart is shown overleaf.

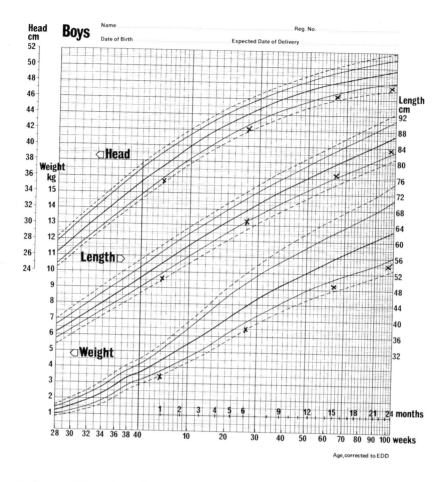

1. Suggest three investigations.
2. What is the diagnosis?

Question 20.2

A 4$\frac{1}{2}$-year-old Bangladeshi boy presented with a 2-week history of jaundice. He had not had any previous episodes, had not recently travelled abroad and he had been generally healthy. His stools were a normal colour and his urine was not dark. He was not taking any medication. There were three siblings who were all well. The parents were first cousins and were also healthy.

On examination he was pale and jaundiced. His liver was enlarged to 3 cm and his spleen was just palpable. His height was 103 cm (25th centile), weight 15.9 kg (10th centile) and examination was otherwise normal.

Haemoglobin	7.6 g/dl
White cell count	$14.2 \times 10^9/l$
Platelet count	$289 \times 10^9/l$
Serum sodium	137 mmol/l
Serum potassium	5.1 mmol/l
Serum urea	4.6 mmol/l
Serum creatinine	54 mmol/l
Serum bilirubin	45 μmol/l
Serum bicarbonate	25 mmol/l
Serum alkaline phosphatase	499 IU/l
Serum alanine transferase	13 IU/l
Serum protein	81 g/l
Serum albumin	50 g/l
Serum iron	17.4 μmol/l (normal 14–25 μmol/l)
Serum ferritin	55 μg/l (normal 15–300 μg/l)
Serum haptoglobin	1.13 μg/l (normal 1–3 μg/l)
Total iron	54 nmol/l (normal 45–80 nmol/l)
Glucose-6-phosphate dehydrogenase	Normal
Hepatitis A and B serology	Negative
Blood film	Marked hypochromia, moderate spherocytosis, moderate aniso-cytosis, marked anisochromia, marked microcytosis, moderate number of target cells

1. What is the diagnosis?
2. What two investigations are required to confirm this?

Question 20.3

A 7-year-old caucasian boy with known juvenile chronic arthritis was admitted with a 2-week history of general malaise, low-grade pyrexia and nausea. Over the last 3 days he had also been complaining of epigastric discomfort and increasing stiffness in his joints. There had been no contact with any illness and he had never been abroad. His arthritis presented 5 months previously and his symptoms were difficult to control. His current medication was benorylate, naproxen and sulphasalazine.

On examination he looked pale and mildly jaundiced, but was apyrexial. He had marked cervical, axillary and inguinal lymphadenopathy. His liver was palpable 4 cm below the costal margin and was non-tender. His spleen was also palpable 2 cm below the costal margin.

Haemoglobin	7.3 g/dl
White cell count	5.6×10^9/l
Platelet count	78×10^9/l
INR	1.8
Total protein	57 g/l
Albumin	39 g/l
Alkaline phophatase	386 IU/l (normal <350 IU/l)
Gamma glutamyl transferase	534 IU/l (normal 5–55 IU/l)
Alanine transaminase	141 IU/l (normal 2–53 IU/l)
Total bilirubin	82 µmol/l

1. Suggest two possible causes for this boy's jaundice.
2. What three investigations would you perform?
3. How would you manage the case further?

Question 20.4

A healthy, well-grown, 4-year-old boy presented with swelling of his right parotid gland over a 2-day period. He had had a mild pyrexia and was more lethagic than usual. Examination revealed pain and tenderness over the distribution of his parotid gland. The gland was difficult to delineate precisely by palpation and the orifice of Stensen's duct appeared red and slightly swollen. The parotid swelling eventually resolved after 8 days. He was noted not to have had his MMR vaccination, and this was given shortly after the end of the illness. A week later he was seen with a cough that had been noted for the past 2–3 weeks but which had become more pronounced. There was a history of tuberculosis in a grandparent so a 1 in 1000 Mantoux test was performed. At 72 h a 3 mm area of induration was seen.

Six months later a similar swelling of the other parotid gland developed, associated with mild pyrexia and malaise. This lasted for 6 days and the parotid gland was tender. Antibiotics were given at the beginning of this episode and had no immediate effect. Eight months later the boy again had an episode in his left parotid gland, which lasted several days. On this occasion purulent fluid could be expressed from the orifice of the parotid duct. He experienced no weight loss during this period of time and his general hygiene was considered to be good. Dental inspection revealed no abnormalities.

1. What is your differential diagnosis?
2. What would your advice be with regard to his Mantoux result?
3. Give two investigations you would perform.

Question 20.5

A 1-year-old boy was admitted as a day case for immunization as he had had rashes thought to be associated with eating eggs. About 30 min following administration of MMR vaccine he developed a sinus tachycardia of 130 beats/min. An intensely itchy rash rapidly developed on his face and body. The rash had raised erythematous edges and was urticarial. He became hypotensive, his blood pressure being 60/25 mmHg.

1. What steps must be taken immediately?

Paper 20 *ANSWERS*

Answer 20.1

1. Full blood count
   Serum metabolic profile
   Stools for ova cysts and parasites
   Stool for culture
   Stool for fat
   Stool for reducing substances

   Differntial sugar test
   Xylose absorption test
   Serum iron

   Anti-gliadin anti-reticulum antibodies

2. Non-specific toddler diarrhoea

Reject: Food allergy
   Coeliac disease

Discussion

This child presents the typical picture of non-specific toddler diarrhoea. The finding of recognizable pieces of food is characteristic. His growth is perfectly adequate and there is a case for undertaking no investigation at this stage. Where tests are performed their purpose is to look for evidence of malabsorption and other causes of persistent diarrhoea, e.g. infection and coeliac disease. In this case there is no information given to support a diagnosis of coeliac disease or food allergy.

Answer 20.2

1. ß-thalassaemia (intermedia or major)
   α-thalassaemia
   Sickle cell disease

   Lead poisoning

Reject: Malaria
   Liver disease
   Iron deficiency
   Spherocytosis (or other haemolytic anaemias)

2. Haemoglobin electrophoresis
Red cell indices

Lead level

Reject: Red cell fragility study

Discussion

The important findings are jaundice, low haemoglobin, normal iron studies, normal haptoglobin and the blood film. Target cells are found in several conditions, but apart from the jaundice his liver function is normal. The low haemoglobin is consistent with sickle cell disease or some other rare haemoglobinopathies. Lead poisoning is possible but unlikely in view of the normal physical examination. A haemolytic anaemia is excluded by the normal haptoglobin and hypochromia. However, from the evidence of the blood film the most likely diagnosis is a thalassaemia. This is confirmed by electrophoresis.

Answer 20.3

1. Infective hepatitis
Drug reaction

2. Hepatitis A/B serology
CMV
Toxoplasmosis and EBV serology
C3, C4, C3d
Serum immunoglobulins

3. Discontinue sulphasalazine and benorylate
Monitor liver function and INR
If continued deterioration, commence high-dose steroids

Reject: Liver biospy

Discussion

It is important to exclude an infective cause for the jaundice as a first step in the management of this case. Liver disease (the nature of which is not entirely clear) is a rare complication of treatment with sulphasalazine. It is associated with an increase in activated T cells and immune complexes, massive hypergammaglobulinaemia and a variable degree of anaemia and thrombocytopenia. Fatalities have been reported. Since benorylate contains paracetamol, it should also be discontinued in this case.

Answer 20.4

1. Recurrent parotitis

Infection with HIV

2. Repeat Mantoux test 4–6 weeks later as initial result may have been a false negative

3. X-ray of parotid gland duct to exclude a stone
Sialograms of both parotid glands
Test for HIV infection

Discussion

Recurrent parotitis of childhood is characterized by rapid and repeated swelling of one or both parotid glands and is accompanied by the symptoms described above. The usual age of onset is between 3 and 6 years and attacks recur at a variable interval up to 8 months. In most cases there is a spontaneous remission of episodes during adolescence. Duration of attacks appears to be independent of antibiotic therapy and the condition is presumed to be non-infectious. First and second episodes are often thought to be examples of suppurative parotitis and accordingly are treated with antimicrobial agents. Parotitis may also be seen as one of the protean manifestations of infection with the human immunodeficiency virus. However, it is a much less likely diagnosis in this situation.

A 1 in 1000 Mantoux test read after 72 h showing 3 mm of induration is a negative finding. However, measles virus inhibits the response to tuberculin, so tuberculin-positive individuals may become tuberculin negative for up to a month after measles infection or MMR vaccine. The Mantoux test should be repeated 4–6 weeks later.

In cases of recurrent parotitis it is appropriate to perform sialography. Prior to sialography a scout film should be taken to scan for the presence of a stone. If a stone is found, sialography is not indicated.

Answer 20.5

1. a   Airway — he should be placed in the left lateral position and airway kept open

     b   Breathing — his ventilatory effort should be assessed and oxygen administered

     c   Circulation — 1 in 10 000 adrenaline (0.1 ml/kg for his age) given by deep intramuscular injection

     d   Call for assistance

     e   Chlorpheniramine maleate and hydrocortisone may be given intravenously and the line left in situ

     f   Administration of intravenous fluid

Discussion

This is a case of anaphylactic reaction to MMR. The basic steps of resuscitation should be performed — airway, breathing and circulation must be assessed and reassessed. As further interventions such as intubation may be necessary, *help* is absolutely vital.

INDEX TO QUESTIONS